Springer-Verlag Berlin Heidelberg GmbH

Springer-Verlag Berlin Heidelberg GmbH

João A. C. Navarro

The Nasal Cavity and Paranasal Sinuses

Surgical Anatomy

Coauthors João de Lima Navarro
Paulo de Lima Navarro

With 150 Color Figures

Springer

João A.C. Navarro
Professor and Chairman of Anatomy
Department of Morphology
Dental School of Bauru
University of São Paulo
Bauru, SP
Brazil

João de Lima Navarro
Graduate in Computer Sciences
Exact Sciences Center
State University of Londrina
Londrina, Paraná
Brazil

Paulo de Lima Navarro
Medical Doctor
Health Sciences Center
State University of Londrina
Londrina, Paraná
Brazil

Translators:

Dr. Márcia Murao
Dr. Suzana M. de Oliveira

Original Edition:
João A.C. Navarro
Cavidade do Nariz e Seios Paranasais
(Anatomia Cirúrgica 1)
© All Dent. (Bauru) 1997

Library of Congress Cataloging-in-Publication Data
Navarro, João A.C. (João Adolfo Caldas), 1939. The nasal cavity and
paranasal sinuses : surgical anatomy / João A.C. Navarro ; [contri-
butor, Paulo de Lima Navarro]. p. ; cm. – (Surgical anatomy).
Includes bibliographical references and index.

1. Nasal fossa–Anatomy. 2. Paranasal sinuses–Anatomy. 3. Anatomy,
Surgical and topographical. I. Navarro, Paulo de Lima. II. Title. III.
Series.
[DNLM: 1. Nasal Cavity–anatomy & histology. 2. Nasal Cavity–sur-
gery. 3. Paranasal Sinuses–anatomy & histology. 4. Paranasal Sinu-
ses–surgery. WV 301 N322n 2001]
QM505 .N385 2001   611'.92–dc21   00-061189

ISBN 978-3-540-67578-5   ISBN 978-3-642-56829-9 (eBook)
DOI 10.1007/978-3-642-56829-9

© Springer-Verlag Berlin Heidelberg 2001
Originally published by Springer-Verlag Berlin Heidelberg
New York in 2001

Cover design: Erich Kirchner, Heidelberg
Typesetting and data conversion of the figures:
AM-productions GmbH, Wiesloch

Printed on acid-free paper   SPIN: 10763870   24/3130/PF
5 4 3 2 1 0

To my wife Fidela,
and to my sons
Paulo, João, Marcos, and Ricardo,
for their love and involvement

Foreword

The evolution of microscopic and endoscopic surgery of the nose was made possible due to the detailed knowledge acquired by anatomists and surgeons on the macro- and microanatomy of this region.

Unveiling the complex structure of the middle third of the face has always been a challenge to Prof. Navarro. The contribution of his studies to the many specialties is immeasurable. The present work comprises information on the main anatomic references of the nose, paranasal sinuses, and related structures, essential for everyone concerned with microendoscopic surgery of the paranasal sinuses.

I would like to thank Prof. Navarro once more for his teachings, which have greatly contributed to my own professional development and to that of so many colleagues all over the world.

Aldo Stamm

Preface

In the field of health sciences, steady and rapid advances in knowledge demand from the professional true commitment and continued efforts to keep abreast of the times. For the medical surgeon, a deep knowledge of basic biology and anatomy becomes more and more necessary, considering the diagnostic advances and the refinement of surgical techniques which have been made possible by the development of novel equipment and modern tools. Since ancient times, a deep understanding of anatomy has stood out as an essential requirement for surgical activities.

The anatomy textbooks and atlases currently available for students and clinicians, many of them dating from previous centuries, are often not up-to-date. They usually lack important information on anatomical variations naturally occurring in individuals, especially those of the deep craniofacial regions. Moreover, specialized publications hardly ever include mesoscopic anatomical preparations (preparations carried out under the surgical microscope), which are useful for microsurgery and endoscopic surgery within several medical specialties.

To fill this gap, information based on the current literature and on our own experience in anatomy acquired over the years has been collected in this publication. This study of the nasal cavity and paranasal sinuses focuses on their osteological aspects, anatomical relationships, and the sites for surgical access to the paranasal sinuses.

Anatomical aspects of the skull and cadaver were analyzed and compared with those in the living, in order to highlight the regions posing an enhanced surgical risk. Notes of surgical relevance are synthetically presented at the end of the text, constituting an overview of the most important anatomical relationships and aiming to provide the reader with a useful and practical guide to microsurgery and endonasal endoscopic surgery.

J. Navarro

Acknowledgements

My deepest recognition and appreciation are offered to my teacher and friend Dr. Aldo C. Stamm, for his vast contribution to the excellence of the anatomic principles applied to microsurgery and endoscopic surgery.

To Prof. Dr. Dagoberto Sottovia Filho, Director of the Bauru School of Dentistry (University of São Paulo), and to Prof. Dr. José Alberto de Souza Freitas, General Director of the Labiopalatal Damages Recovery Hospital (University of São Paulo), for their encouragement and support of our projects and myself; to my sons Paulo de Lima Navarro and João de Lima Navarro, who, with much personal effort, contributed greatly to the preparation of the manuscript; to Dr. Regina Célia Baptista Belluzzo, Technical Director of the Library and Documentation Service, and to Eliane Falcão Tuler Xavier, Technical Head of the Library Service of Documentation and Publicity of the Bauru School of Dentistry, (University of São Paulo), for their excellent job and unselfish dedication. To each I extend my deepest appreciation.

To my colleagues Prof. Dr. Neivo Luiz Zorzetto, João Lopes Toledo Filho, and Jesus Carlos Andrêo, for their supportive collaboration; to the researchers Regina Papassoni Santos, Érica A.P. Oliveira, and Silmara Valderez Zamboni; to the members of our staff Mr. Orivaldo da Silva, Mr. Romário M. de Arruda, and Ms. Eugênia D. Meggiato, for their permanent interest; to Cláudia V. de Oliveira and Gislene S. de Moraes, for their diligence and unfailing efficiency. I extend my special recognition to all of them and hope we will continue to work together.

To the staff of the City Hall, the Centrinho, and the FOB, who were collaborative and helpful throughout.

To the Brazilian and foreign otorhinolaryngologists with whom I have had the opportunity to work.

To the Brazilian Society of Otorhinolaryngology and the Brazilian Society of Rhinology and Esthetic Facial Surgery, for the qualified support they gave to our enterprise.

To Drs. Eulália Sakano, Elizabeth Araújo Pereira, Rainer Haetinger, Antônio Douglas Menon, Alexandre Fellippu, Roberto M. Neves Pinto, Carlos Alberto H. Campos, Lídio Granato, Pedro O. Cavalcanti, Antônio Carlos Cedin, José Francisco Chagas, Nelson Caldas, and Washington Luiz C. Almeida, for their encouragement and friendship.

To the Otorhinolaryngology and Phonoaudiology Center (COF) and to the Edmundo Vasconcelos Hospital, for the opportunity to participate in the microsurgery and endonasal endoscopic surgery courses over so many years, under the supervision of Dr. Aldo Stamm.

To Doc Med, for their kind support and friendship; to Byk Química, for their permanent commitment to scientific development, and to Richards do Brasil for their immeasurable help and encouragement.

The participation of so many valuable people has been crucial to the undertaking of this project. To all, my sincerest gratitude.

My special thanks go to Dr. Suzana Macedo de Oliveira and Dr. Márcia Murao, for their translation of this book into the English language.

Contents

Chapter 1   Development and Growth
of the Nasal Cavity
and Paranasal Sinuses   1

Chapter 2   Anterior Aperture of the Nasal Cavity   25

Chapter 3   Posterior Aperture of the Nasal Cavity   31

Chapter 4   Lateral Wall of the Nasal Cavity   37

Chapter 5   Nasal Septum   55

Chapter 6   Arteries and Nerves of the Nasal Cavity
and Paranasal Sinuses   61

Chapter 7   Maxillary Sinus   71

Chapter 8   Frontal Sinus   83

Chapter 9   Ethmoidal Sinus   93

Chapter 10   Sphenoidal Sinus   105

Chapter 11   Cranial Base and Paranasal Sinuses   115

Chapter 12   Notes of Anatomosurgical Importance   125

Recommended Reading   135

Subject Index   141

Chapter 1
Development and Growth of the Nasal Cavity and Paranasal Sinuses

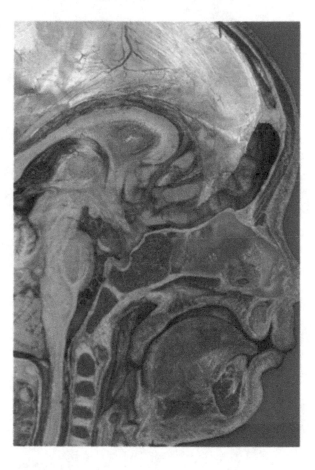

Chapter 1 _____
Development and Growth
of the Nasal Cavity
and Paranasal Sinuses

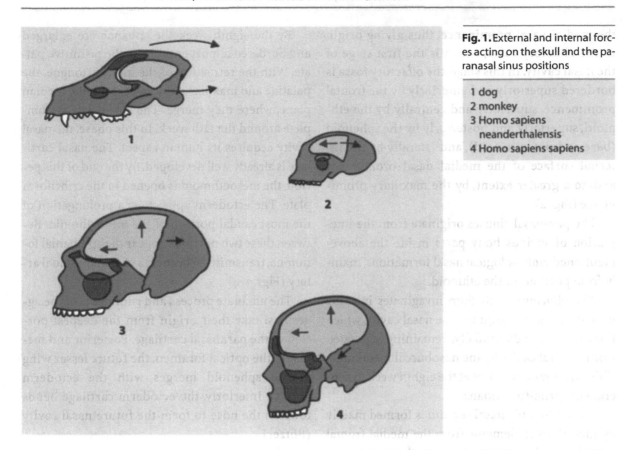

Fig. 1. External and internal forces acting on the skull and the paranasal sinus positions

1 dog
2 monkey
3 Homo sapiens neanderthalensis
4 Homo sapiens sapiens

With the humanization of the primates during evolution, the nose lost its near relation to the mandible and the olfactory sense was reduced. With the retraction of the snout, the verticalization and enlargement of the face, and the orbits migrating anteriorly, the nasal cavity and the paranasal sinuses ended up occupying the interorbital space under the anterior skull and over the oral cavity. The ethmoid became multicellular and expanded laterally, helping to build up the lateral walls of the nasal cavity and participating more intensively in the respiratory process (Fig. 1).

The nose and paranasal sinuses appear to not yet have reached a stable evolutionary condition. Morphofunctional adaptations are still occurring, and the frequent anatomical variations found in this region corroborate this idea. Some aspects of the development and growth of the craniofacial structures require further study for a better understanding of the frequent and numerous changes in this complex anatomical region.

In the 6-week human embryo, a number of prominences that have developed from the neuro- and viscerocranium are already found. In the median sagittal plane, the frontal prominence is divided by the interhemispheric slot, giving rise to both cerebral hemispheres. Immediately below, we may observe both the lateral and medial nasal prominences, as well as the globular process located over the primitive mouth, whose boundaries are the maxillary and mandibular processes of the first branchial arch.

In this stage, the rough draft of the nasal cavity is represented by two furrows at either side of the frontal bone, between the medial, globular, and lateral nasal prominences. The ectoderm thickens to generate the olfactory epithelium. The maxillary prominences project themselves very rapidly towards the median line, occupying a position under the lateral nasal prominence, binding to it and obliterating the orbitonasal slot. Simultaneously, they also bind to the lateral end of the medial nasal prominence, thus giving origin to the olfactory fossa, which is the first stage of the nasal cavity. In this stage, the olfactory fossa is bordered superiorly and anteriorly by the frontal prominence, superiorly and centrally by the ethmoid, superiorly and posteriorly by the sphenoid (base and pre-sphenoid), and laterally by the internal surface of the medial nasal prominence and, to a greater extent, by the maxillary prominence (Fig. 2).

The paranasal sinuses originate from the integration of various bony parts inside the above-mentioned embryological nasal formations, mainly from portions of the ethmoid.

The olfactory epithelium invaginates into the mesoderm, giving origin to the nasal cavity, which thereafter extends caudally, remaining separated from the oral cavity by the nasobuccal membrane. This membrane ruptures at the eighth week to generate the primitive choanae.

The embryonic nasal septum is formed mainly by mesodermic elements from the medial frontal prominence. It is situated between the nostrils and binds to the palatine and pterygopalatine plates. By the fifth week, the primitive nasobuccal membrane ruptures, connecting the choanae with the primitive oral cavity. The nasolacrimal duct is formed between the maxillary and the lateral nasal prominences. Following the rupture of the nasobuccal membrane, the primitive nasal cavity remains bordered on each side by a cavity that opens anteriorly as the nostrils and posteriorly as the primitive choanae.

By the eighth week the choanae are enlarged and bordered almost entirely by the primitive palate. With the retraction of the inferior tongue, the palatine and maxillary processes reach the median plane, where they merge. The soft palate is complete around the 12th week. In this phase, the nasal cavity acquires its human aspect. The nasal cartilage is already well developed. By the end of this period, the mesoethmoid is opened in the cribriform plate. The ectoderm appears as a prolongation of the most caudal portion of the mesoethmoid. Between these two portions appear the epiphanial foramina, transmitting branches of the ethmoidal artery (Figs. 3, 4).

The uncinate process and rudiments of the agger nasi take their origin from the deepest portion of the paranasal cartilage. Posterior and medial to the optical foramen, the future lesser wing of the sphenoid merges with the ectoderm (Fig. 5). Inferiorly, the ectoderm cartilage bends towards the nose to form the future nasal cavity (Blitzer).

Fig. 2. Six-week human embryo, anterior view. Processes

1. frontonasal	10. cerebral hemisphere
2. median nasal	11. nasal cavity roof
3. lateral frontal	12. nasal cavity opening
4. lateral nasal	13. palatine fossa
5. globular (eye)	14. primitive mouth
6. nasolacrimal duct	15. intermaxillary
7. maxillary process	incisura
8. mandibular process	16. second branchial
9. interhemispherical	arch
incisura	

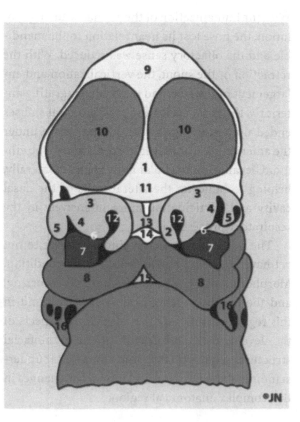

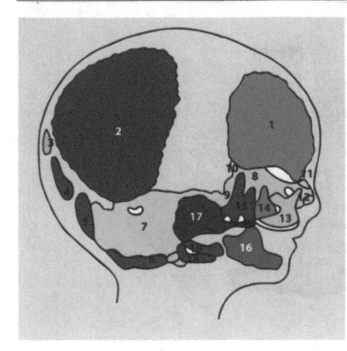

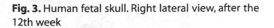

Fig. 3. Human fetal skull. Right lateral view, after the 12th week

1. frontal
2. parietal
3. pre-interparietal
4. interparietal
5. supraoccipital
6. exo-occipital
7. auditory cartilaginous capsule
8. ethmoid (nasal cartilaginous capsule)
9. sphenoidal base
10. pre-sphenoid
11. nasal
12. lacrimal
13. maxilla
14. zygomatic
15. sphenoidal greater wing
16. Meckel's cartilage
17. temporal
18. vaginal process
19. tympanic bone

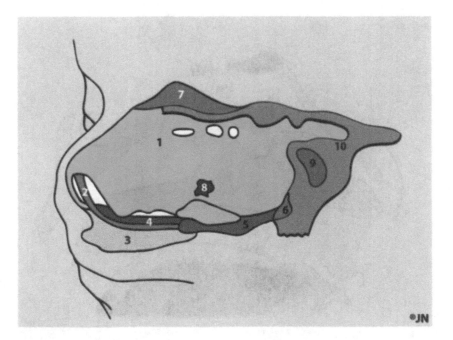

Fig. 4. Nasal cartilaginous capsule of a 16-week human fetus

1. nasal capsule	4. paraseptal cartilage	7. crista galli	10. sphenoidal lesser wing
2. nasal septum	5. vomer	8. lacrimal	
3. maxilla	6. palatine	9. optic canal	

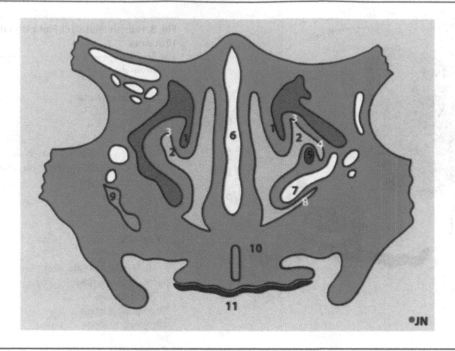

Fig. 5. Nasal cavity, coronal cut at the nasal middle meatus of a 14-week human fetus

1. middle nasal concha	4. maxillary sinus	7. inferior nasal concha	10. palatine suture
2. middle nasal meatus	5. uncinate process	8. inferior nasal meatus	11. palatine papilla
3. frontal recess	6. nasal septum	9. nasolacrimal duct	

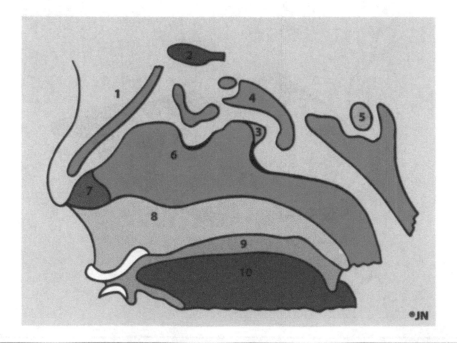

Fig. 6. Nasal cavity, sagittal cut of a 12-week human fetus

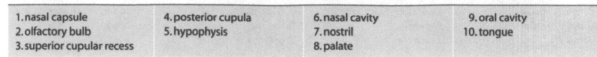

1. nasal capsule	4. posterior cupula	6. nasal cavity	9. oral cavity
2. olfactory bulb	5. hypophysis	7. nostril	10. tongue
3. superior cupular recess		8. palate	

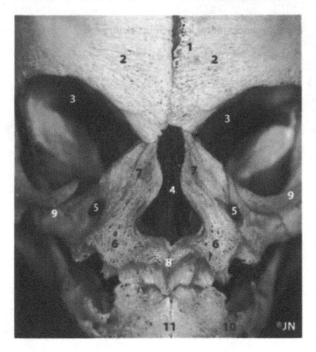

Fig. 7. Anterior view of a 16-week human fetal skull

1. interfrontal suture (metopic)	7. frontal process
2. frontal	8. alveolar process
3. orbit	9. zygomatic
4. nasal cavity	10. mandible
5. infraorbital foramen	11. mandibular symphysis
6. maxilla	

The epithelium of the nasal cavity proliferates by invaginating deeply in the connective tissue of the nasal wall, provoking ruptures in some parts of the embryonic mesenchyma. The future nasal conchae are thus formed, remaining lined by a tissue which is in fact an extension of the epithelium of the nasal cavity.

The inferior nasal concha (maxilloturbinal concha) appears as an elongated prominence anterior to the choanae. The inferior nasal meatus, still narrow in the newborn, becomes progressively concave at the nasal side and convex at the side of the maxillary sinus. At the same time, an identical projection appears over the inferior nasal concha, which will be the first ethmoidal (maxilloethmoidal) concha. A second or a third ethmoidal concha will successively appear over this one, growing towards the septum. The concave spaces between them at the nasal lateral wall are known as nasal meatus. The third ethmoidal concha, called the supreme (Santorini), may occur in the posterosuperior angle of the nasal cavity. The ethmoidal conchae may display grooves, corresponding to the divisions named the secondary nasal conchae by Zuckerkandl.

The middle meatus becomes deeply grooved and generates the infundibulum, from which the uncinate process, a secondary nasal concha, stands out. Dorsal to the infundibulum some other grooves appear, delimiting other secondary nasal conchae. The ethmoidal bulla is generated by the fusion of two secondary nasal conchae and constitutes the dorsal boundary of the infundibulum, thus forming the embryonic infundibular sac, which in turn will become the semilunar hiatus. A groove appears in the superior portion of the maxilloturbinal concha (inferior nasal concha), which will be pneumatized and will protrude into the lateral wall of the nasal cavity as the agger nasi.

The epithelial slot formed between the maxilloturbinal and ethmoidoturbinal conchae will be the middle nasal meatus, which is a region of great functional importance, the origin of most of the paranasal sinuses (Figs. 11, 12).

The maxillary and frontal processes and the anterior ethmoidal cells protrude from the embryonic infundibulum (van Alyea). The maxillary sinus appears in the early fetal stage, around the 12th week, in the form of a small invagination starting at the infundibulum. The infundibular prolongation extends superiorly and anteriorly as the frontal recess. The anterior ethmoidal cells will originate from the superior and posterior borders of the frontal recess. At birth, the ethmoidal portion between the cribriform plate and the middle nasal concha is twice the size of the maxillary portion. In the adult, these two portions are equal in size. The nasal common meatus is narrow in the newborn, making respiration difficult; this may lead to mucosal congestion and eventually to a pathological condition (Fig. 7–10).

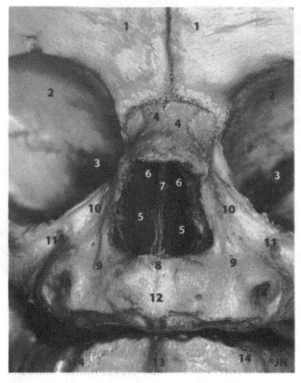

Fig. 8. Anterior view of a newborn's skull

1. frontal	8. anterior nasal spine
2. orbit	9. maxilla
3. superior orbital fissure	10. frontal process
4. nasal	11. infraorbital foramen
5. nasal cavity	12. intermaxillary suture
6. middle nasal concha	13. mandible
7. nasal septum	14. dental buds

Fig. 9. Anterior view of a 1-year-old child's skull

1. frontal	11. intermaxillary suture
2. nasal	12. dental buds in the maxilla
3. orbit	13. deciduous maxillary incisors
4. superior orbital fissure	14. deciduous inferior incisors
5. optic foramen	15. mandible
6. infraorbital foramen	16. dental buds in the mandible
7. maxilla	
8. nasal cavity	
9. nasal septum	
10. middle nasal concha	

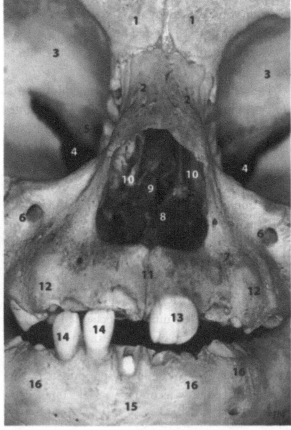

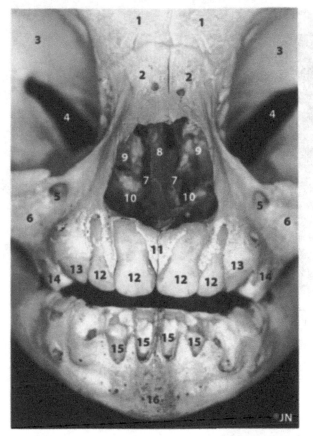

Fig. 10. Anterior view of an 18-month-old child's skull

1. frontal	11. intermaxillary suture
2. nasal	12. deciduous maxillary
3. orbit	incisors
4. superior orbital fissure	13. deciduous canine
5. infraorbital foramen	14. maxillary deciduous
6. maxilla	first molar
7. nasal cavity	15. deciduous inferior
8. nasal septum	incisors
9. middle nasal concha	16. mandible
10. inferior nasal concha	

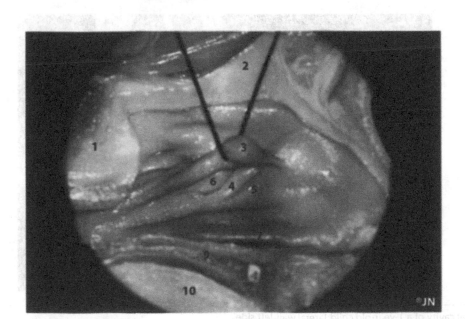

Fig. 11. Sagittal cut of a 14-week human fetal head, left side

1. cartilaginous sphenoid	3. reflected middle	5. middle nasal meatus	8. inferior nasal meatus
2. cartilaginous crista galli	nasal concha	6. ethmoidal bulla	9. palate
	4. uncinate process	7. inferior nasal concha	10. tongue

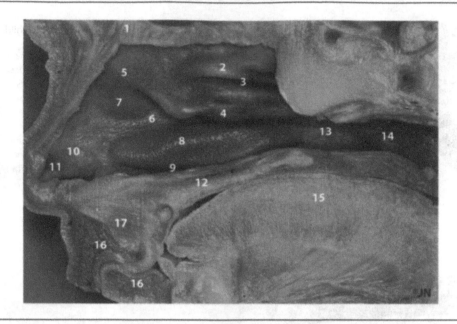

Fig. 12. Nasal cavity of a 16-week human fetus, lateral wall, right side

1. crista galli	6. middle nasal meatus	9. inferior nasal meatus	14. nasopharynx
2. superior nasal concha	7. middle nasal meatus	10. limen nasi	15. tongue
3. superior nasal meatus	aditus	11. nostril	16. lips
4. middle nasal concha	8. inferior nasal concha	12. palate	17. dental germ
5. agger nasi		13. choanal region	

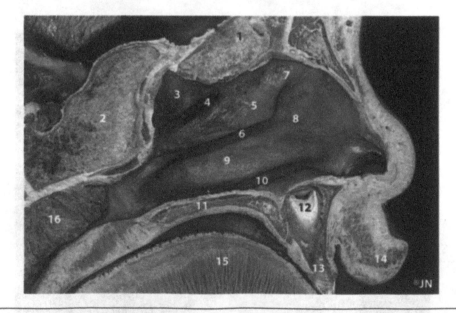

Fig. 13. Nasal cavity of a 1-year-old child, lateral wall, left side

1. crista galli	6. middle nasal meatus	10. inferior nasal meatus	14. superior lip
2. sphenoid	7. agger nasi	11. palate	15. tongue
3. superior nasal concha	8. middle nasal meatus aditus	12. dental germ (permanent)	16. adenoid
4. superior nasal meatus	9. inferior nasal concha	13. deciduous maxillary	
5. middle nasal concha		incisor	

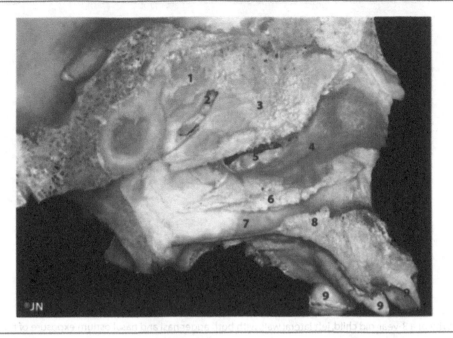

Fig. 14. Nasal cavity of a 5-year-old child, bony lateral wall, left side

1. superior nasal concha	4. middle nasal meatus	6. inferior nasal concha	8. palate
2. superior nasal meatus	5. maxillary window	7. inferior nasal meatus	9. deciduous teeth
3. middle nasal concha			

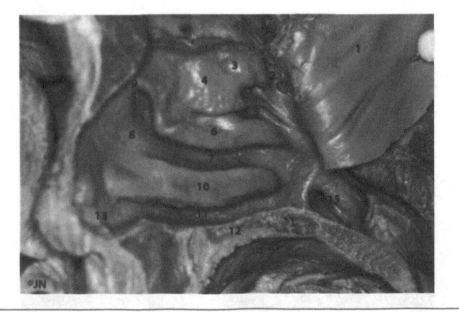

Fig. 15. Nasal cavity of a 3-year-old child, right lateral wall

1. nasal septum (reflected)	5. superior nasal meatus	9. agger nasi region	14. oral cavity
2. ostium of sphenoidal sinus	6. middle nasal concha	10. inferior nasal concha	15. pharyngeal opening of auditory tube
3. supreme nasal concha	7. middle nasal meatus	11. inferior nasal meatus	
4. superior nasal concha	8. aditus of middle nasal meatus	12. palate	
		13. nostril	

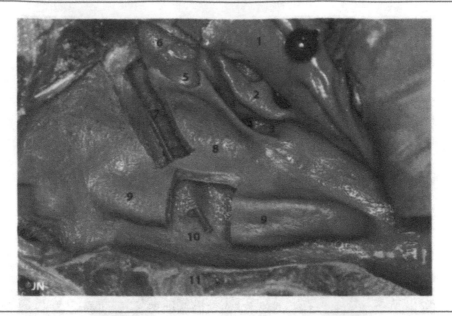

Fig. 16. Nasal cavity of a 3-year-old child, left lateral wall, with both agger nasi and nasal ostium exposure of nasolacrimal duct

1. reflected middle nasal concha	5. uncinate process, pneumatized by agger nasi cell	7. nasal wall of nasolacrimal duct	9. sectioned inferior nasal concha, showing ostium of the nasolacrimal duct (with probe)
2. ethmoidal bulla	6. agger nasi cell	8. middle nasal meatus	
3. maxillary sinus ostium			10. inferior nasal meatus
4. semilunar hiatus			11. palate

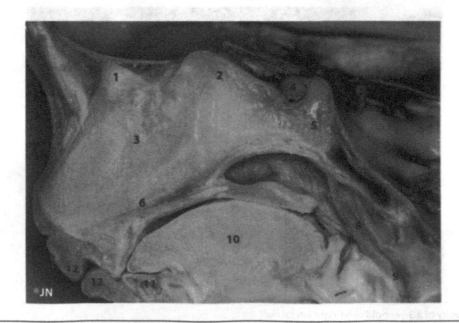

Fig. 17. Nasal septum of a 16-week human fetus, left side

1. crista galli	4. hypophyseal fossa	7. nasopharynx	10. tongue
2. pre-sphenoid	5. basal portion of sphenoid	8. oropharynx	11. dental germ
3. nasal cartilaginous septum	6. palate	9. laryngopharynx	12. lips

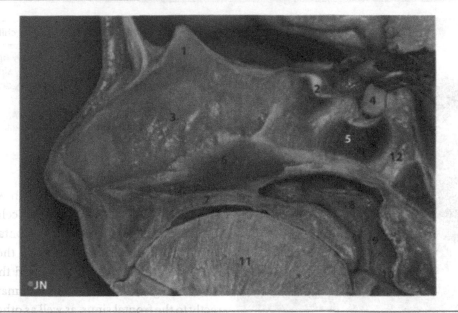

Fig. 18. Nasal septum of a 20-week human fetus, left side

1. crista galli	4. hypophyseal fossa	8. nasopharynx	12. spheno-occipital
2. pre-sphenoid	5. basal portion of sphenoid	9. oropharynx	synchondrosis
3. nasal cartilaginous	6. vomer	10. laryngopharynx	
septum	7. palate	11. tongue	

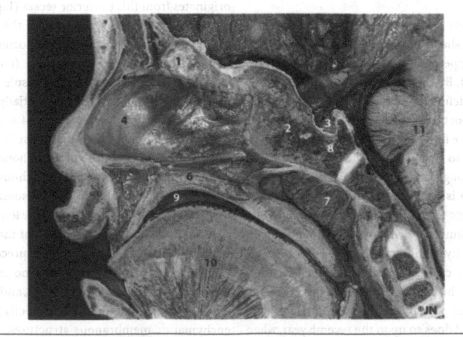

Fig. 19. Nasal septum of a 1-year-old child, right side

1. crista galli	4. nasal septum	7. adenoid	9. oral cavity
2. sphenoid	5. lip	8. spheno-occipital	10. tongue
3. hypophyseal fossa	6. palate	synchondrosis	11. brain stem

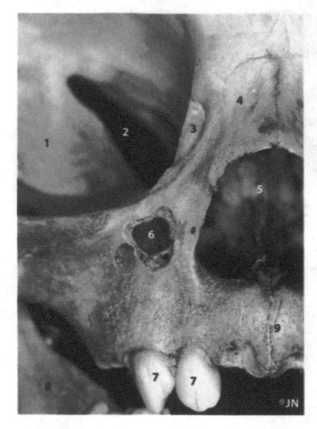

Fig. 20. Bony maxillary sinus of a 2-year-old child

1. orbit	6. anteriorly opened
2. superior orbital fissure	maxillary sinus
3. lacrimal fossa	7. maxillary deciduous
4. nasal	teeth
5. nasal cavity	8. mandible
	9. intermaxillary suture

At birth, the maxillary sinus presents as a round or elongated shape, becoming gradually pyramidal with the appearance of the permanent teeth (Figs. 20–22). By the 13th year the maxillary sinus reaches its definitive shape, and around the 18th year its proportions are stable.

During the first fetal months, the nasal cavity is very similar to that in the adult. Every element is present, although in a very reduced size. The fourth nasal concha is commonly found until birth, after which it starts to recede due to the growth of the posterior ethmoidal cells towards the interior of the nasal cavity. Until birth, the nasal septum is almost entirely cartilaginous, except for the region occupied by the growing vomer. At this stage, the perpendicular plate of the ethmoid starts growing vertically and does so up to the seventh year, when it becomes appositional. By the 12th or 13th year the septum acquires its definitive aspect (Figs. 18, 19).

By the 13th year the maxillary sinus reaches its definitive shape and around the 18th year its pro-

portions are stable. Around the 13th week, one of the three or four ethmoidofrontal cells penetrate into the frontal bone to form the frontal sinus. The other cells will contribute to form the ethmoidal bulla, the middle nasal concha, and the uncinate-lacrimal region. The infundibulum may extend directly to the frontal sinus, as well as other cells originating from the bulla, the uncinate process, the lacrimal region, or from the middle nasal concha itself (van Alyea).

In the 12-week human fetus, the posterior portion of the cartilaginous nasal capsule is completely separated from the basal plate (the precursor cartilage of the sphenoid). The sphenoidal sinus originates from this posterior recess (Fig. 6).

In this first embryonic stage, the primitive sphenoidal sinus is located in the posterior cavity of the nasal cartilaginous capsule (cupulate recess); in a second stage, a bony capsule covers the cartilaginous one, and then is partially resorbed in preparation for the formation of a sphenoidal sinus independent of the nasal capsule. In the last stage, the pneumatization of the sphenoidal sinus occurs. This phase lasts until adulthood (Figs. 13, 15, 32). The nasal and auditory capsules turn into osseous structures. The base and the lesser wing of the sphenoid, the petrous portion of the temporal bone, and the occipital bone are preceded by a cartilaginous template. The frontal bone, the squamous portion of the temporal bone, and the greater wings of the sphenoid derive directly from mesenchymal or membranous structures. The cartilage of the first branchial arch, represented by the maxillary prominence, will contribute to form the nasal cavity. The maxillary prominence will delimit the nasal cavity and the maxillary sinus

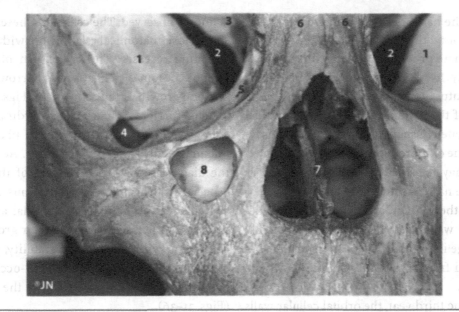

Fig. 21. Bony maxillary sinus of a 5-year-old child

1. orbit	4. inferior orbital fissure	6. nasal bone	8. anteriorly opened
2. superior orbital fissure	5. lacrimal fossa	7. nasal cavity	maxillary sinus
3. optic foramen			

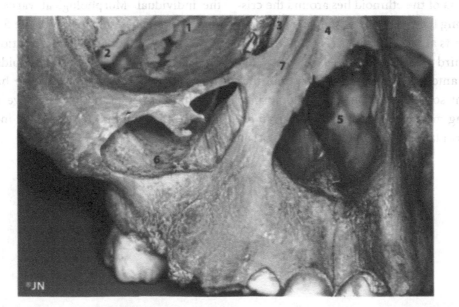

Fig. 22. Bony maxillary sinus of a 7-year-old child

1. orbit	4. nasal bone	6. anteriorly opened	7. frontal maxillary
2. inferior orbital fissure	5. nasal cavity	maxillary sinus	process
3. lacrimal fossa			

(Figs. 3–5). The nasal cavity becomes anatomically defined around the third fetal week.

The uncinate process is prolonged posteriorly and inferiorly from the agger nasi to under the semilunar hiatus, which is relatively wider due to the growth of the ethmoidal bulla. The ethmoidal bulla is elongated in shape, as is the lateral sinus lying over it. One or more accessory ostia of the maxillary sinus may be present, always in the free areas of the middle nasal meatus (see Figs. 29, 30, 34).

At birth, the ethmoidal cells present well-defined orbital walls, near the medial orbital wall. They are large in number but small in volume, being separated from the orbit by a thin bony plate (Figs. 23–26).

Around the third year, the orbital cellular walls of the ethmoid are already tied to the orbit. Because at this age the maxillary sinus has not yet reached its adult proportions, a bony ridge remains between them and the orbitomaxillary border (Figs. 24, 25).

In the newborn, the cranial surfaces of the ethmoidal cells are still separated from the anterior cranial base by a 4- to 8-mm bony plate. The cribriform lamina of the ethmoid lies around the crista galli, among the cellular sets. In the newborn, all these elements are cartilaginous (Figs. 17, 18).

By the third year, the ethmoidal cells are rather close to the anterior cranial base. At this time, they even present some expansion to the supraorbital region, being much more voluminous than in the first year. Frontal and sphenoidal pneumatization is not yet observed. The cells near these areas present a close anatomical relationship with the corresponding recesses. The cribriform plate of the ethmoid becomes elongated and narrow due to the bilateral growth of the cellular set (Figs. 27, 28).

The Torrigiani diagrams, according to Terracol and Ardouin, show the growth phases of the maxillary and sphenoidal sinuses. According to the diagrams, the growth bursts of the sinuses, especially those of the maxillary sinus, are related to dental eruptions. The sphenoidal and frontal sinuses, in turn, seem to have their growth burst coinciding with craniofacial stability, which occurs with the fusion of the spheno-occipital synchondrosis between the 18th and the 20th year (Figs. 31–36).

The growth of the anterior and posterior fossae of the base of the cranium is centered on the sphenoid and ethmoid bones, with which all the neural and visceral bony architecture is anatomically and functionally related. The direct and indirect articulations of these elements, from the early embryonic stage to childhood and adulthood, are fundamental in determining the constitutional type of the individual. Morphological variations occurring before the establishment of the final anatomy may result in craniofacial malformation. An example is nasal obstruction by the adenoids (Fig. 19) or other interferences, leading to the habit of oral breathing. In a period of effective craniofacial growth, this condition may result in malformations.

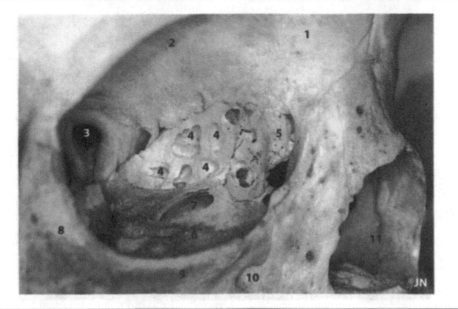

Fig. 23. Bony skull of an 18-month-old child showing the orbit, right side

1. frontal	4. ethmoidal cells	6. inferior orbital wall	9. maxilla
2. superior orbital wall	with orbital walls removed	7. maxillary sinus	10. infraorbital foramen
3. optic foramen	5. lacrimal	8. zygomatic	11. nasal cavity

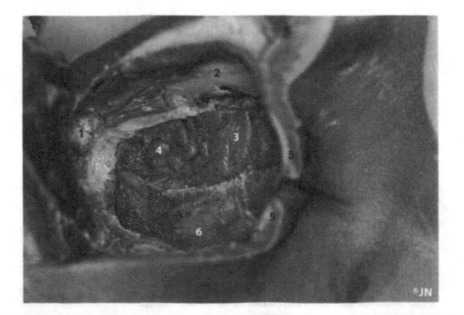

Fig. 24. Ethmoidal cells dissected in the orbit, 1-year-old child, right side

1. optic nerve, sectioned	3. group of anterior	4. group of posterior	5. eyelid
2. superior orbital wall	ethmoidal cells	ethmoidal cells	6. inferior orbital wall

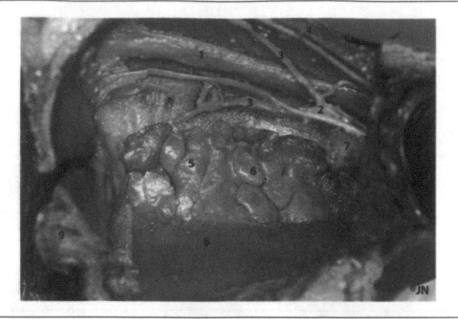

Fig. 25. Orbitally dissected ethmoidal cells, 3-year-old child

1. superior oblique muscle	3. ethmoidal branches of ophthalmic artery	5. group of anterior ethmoidal cells	7. sectioned optic nerve
2. ophthalmic artery	4. frontal nerve	6. group of posterior ethmoidal cells	8. inferior orbital wall
			9. eyelid

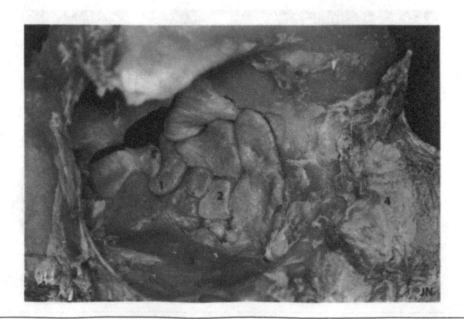

Fig. 26. Orbitally dissected ethmoidal cells in the adult

1. posterior group of ethmoidal cells	2. anterior group of ethmoidal cells	3. inferior orbital wall	4. external nose

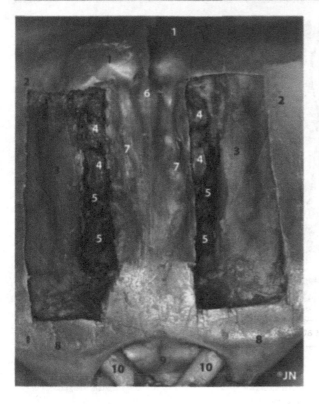

Fig. 27. Ethmoidal cells dissected through the anterior base of the cranium, 1-year-old child

1. endocranial frontal region	6. crista galli
2. frontal orbital lamina	7. ethmoidal cribriform plate
3. periorbita	8. lesser wing of the sphenoid
4. group of anterior ethmoidal cells	9. hypophyseal fossa
5. group of posterior ethmoidal cells	10. optic nerve

Fig. 28. Ethmoidal cells dissected through the anterior base of the cranium, 3-year-old child

1. endocranial frontal region	5. group of posterior ethmoidal cells
2. frontal orbital lamina	6. crista galli
3. periorbita	7. ethmoidal cribriform plate
4. group of anterior ethmoidal cells	

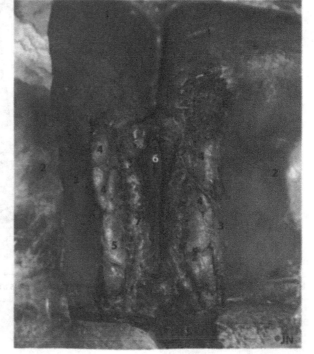

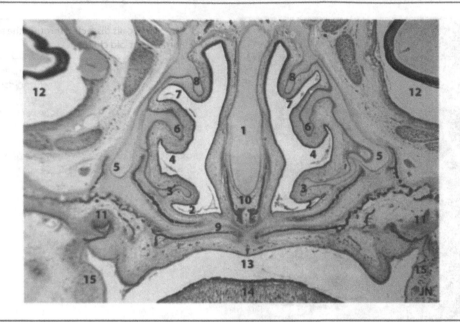

Fig. 29. Histological view of the head of a 16-week human fetus at the posterior level of the nasal cavity (Masson)

1. nasal septum	5. maxillary sinus	9. palate	13. oral cavity
2. inferior nasal meatus	6. middle nasal concha	10. vomer	14. tongue
3. inferior nasal concha	7. superior nasal meatus	11. dental germ	15. buccinator muscle
4. middle nasal meatus	8. superior nasal concha	12. orbit	

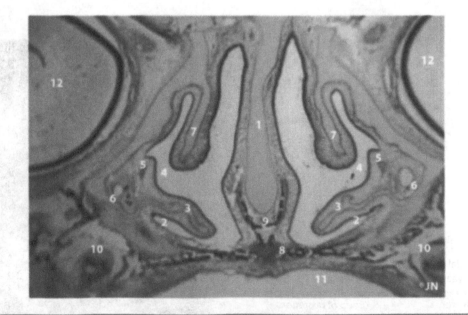

Fig. 30. Histological view of the head of a 16-week human fetus at the median level of the nasal cavity (Masson)

1. nasal septum	4. middle nasal meatus	7. middle nasal concha	10. dental germ
2. inferior nasal meatus	5. uncinate process	8. palate	11. oral cavity
3. inferior nasal concha	6. maxillary sinus	9. vomer	12. orbit

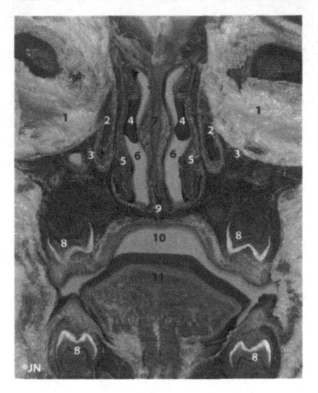

Fig. 31. Coronal section of a 1-year-old child's head, at the middle level of the nasal cavity

1. orbit	7. nasal septum
2. nasolacrimal duct	8. germ of deciduous
3. maxillary sinus	molar
4. middle nasal concha	9. palate
5. inferior nasal concha	10. oral cavity
6. nasal common meatus	11. tongue

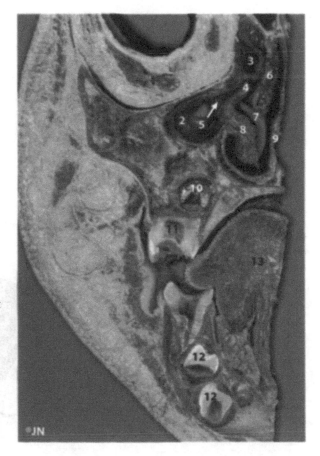

Fig. 32. Coronal view of the hemi-head of a 4-year-old child, at the second deciduous molar level

1. orbit	7. middle nasal meatus
2. maxillary sinus	8. inferior nasal concha
3. ethmoidal bulla	9. nasal septum
4. uncinate process	10. dental germ
5. maxillary sinus duct	11. deciduous molar teeth
and ostium (arrow)	12. premolar teeth
6. middle nasal concha	13. tongue

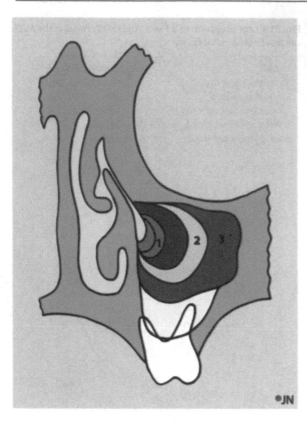

Fig. 33. Diagram of growth of the maxillary sinus from newborn to adult

| 1. in the newborn | 3. in the adult |
| 2. at 12 years of age | |

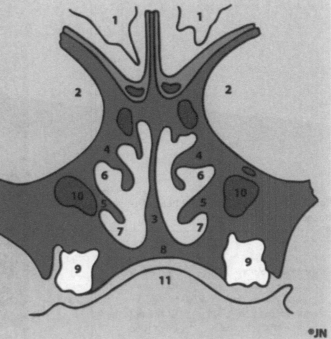

Fig. 34. Schematic coronal view of the head of a 20-week human fetus, at the level of the nasal cavity middle

1. cerebral hemisphere
2. orbit
3. nasal septum
4. middle nasal concha
5. inferior nasal concha
6. middle nasal meatus
7. inferior nasal meatus
8. palate
9. dental germ
10. maxillary sinus
11. oral cavity

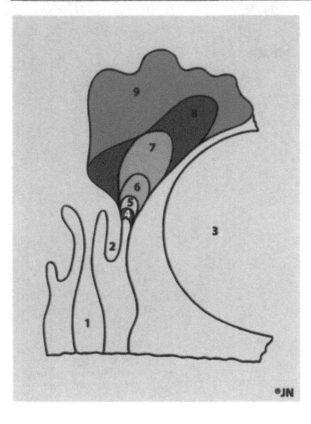

Fig. 35. Growth diagram of the frontal sinus

1. nasal septum	6. at 4 years
2. middle nasal concha	7. at 7 years
3. orbit	8. at 12 years
4. in the newborn	9. in the adult
5. at 1 year	

Fig. 36. Growth diagram of the sphenoidal sinus

1. in the newborn
2. at 3 years
3. at 5 years
4. at 7 years
5. at 12 years
6. in the adult
7. pre-sphenoid

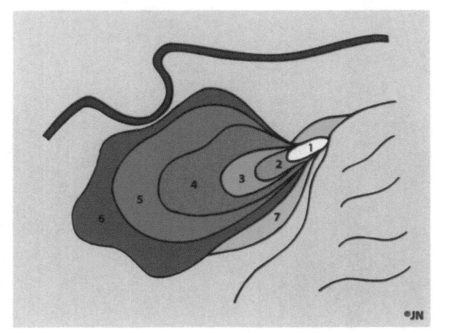

Chapter 2

Anterior Aperture
of the Nasal Cavity

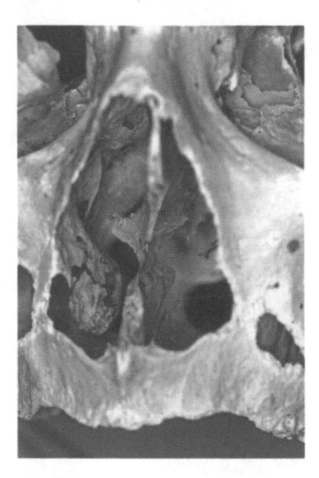

Chapter 2
Anterior Aperture
of the Nasal Cavity

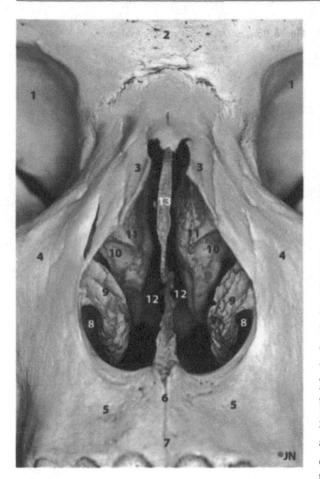

Fig. 37. Bony anterior aperture of nasal cavity

1. orbit	8. inferior nasal meatus
2. frontal	9. inferior nasal concha
3. nasal	10. middle nasal meatus
4. frontal process	11. middle nasal concha
5. alveolar process	12. common nasal meatus
6. anterior nasal spine	13. nasal septum
7. intermaxillary suture	

The base of insertion of the external nose is the anterior bony opening known as the piriform aperture, which is bordered by the nasal and the maxillary frontal processes.

The intermaxillary and internasal sutures either are in the median sagittal plane or deviate slightly from it. The anterior nasal spine is at the most anterior point of the maxillary junction. The nasal and maxillary anterior edges are laminar and somewhat irregular. They define the shape and the width of the piriform aperture, which varies according to race, sex, and age, moreover, it is frequently exposed to traumas, growth malformations, and disease. The range of movement and expansion of the external nose, with its connective, muscular, vasculonervous, and cartilaginous structures comprised into a rigid bony structure, are governed by the sphincter of the nasal limen.

The piriform aperture is divided by the nasal septum, an osteocartilaginous and mucous formation, generally positioned in a paramedian sagittal plane. The bony portion of the septum is formed by the perpendicular plate of the ethmoid and by the vomer. These two structures articulate diagonally, posteroanteriorly and superoinferiorly. The concave anterior edge formed by these laminar bones articulates with the (also laminar) septal cartilage as a prolongation of both bones in the same plane. An intumescence may be seen both in the cadaver and in the living at the junction of the two septal bones with the cartilage (Zuckerkandl), where the septal vasculonervous ends are concentrated.

From the bony lateral wall of the nasal cavity protrude the inferior, the middle, and the superior nasal conchae. Intervening between the conchae, in order of decreasing volume, are the inferior, middle, and superior meatus. Between the nasal septum and the nasal ends of the conchae and meatus is the common nasal meatus (Fig. 37).

The anatomy of the nasal cavity and the varying aerial space within it depend on the position of the nasal septum and on the bony projections in the cavity (Figs. 40–42). In cases of conchal hypertrophy, excessive pneumatization, and septal hypertrophy or deviation, the meatus may be reduced, causing morphofunctional problems. Note that a respiratory mucous connective tissue lines the whole bony skeleton, rendering all nasal structures quite variable in volume (Fig. 38).

The aditus of the nasal cavity is bordered laterally by the frontal maxillary processes, used by surgeons as a guide and a rest for surgical instruments

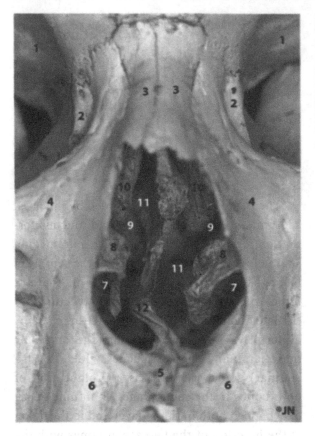

Fig. 38. Bony anterior aperture of nasal cavity

1. orbit	8. inferior nasal concha
2. lacrimal	9. middle nasal meatus
3. nasal	10. middle nasal concha
4. frontal process	11. common nasal meatus
5. anterior nasal spine	12. nasal septum,
6. alveolar process	with right deviation
7. inferior nasal meatus	

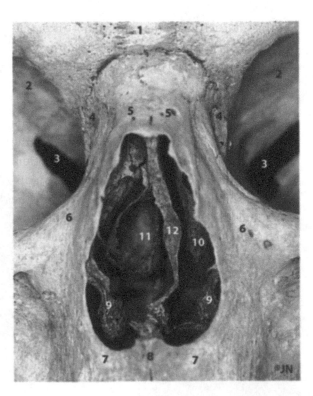

Fig. 39. Bony anterior aperture of nasal cavity

1. frontal	8. anterior nasal spine
2. orbit	9. inferior nasal concha
3. superior orbital fissure	10. middle nasal concha
4. lacrimal	11. middle bullous nasal
5. nasal	concha
6. frontal process	12. nasal septum,
7. alveolar process	with left deviation

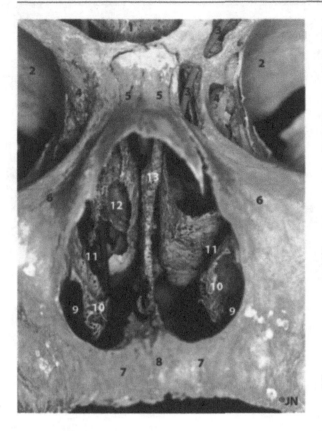

Fig. 40. Bony anterior aperture of nasal cavity

1. frontal sinus	8. anterior nasal spine
2. orbit	9. inferior nasal meatus
3. anterior ethmoidal cell	10. inferior nasal concha
4. lacrimal	11. middle nasal meatus
5. nasal	12. middle bullous nasal
6. frontal process	concha
7. alveolar process	13. nasal septum

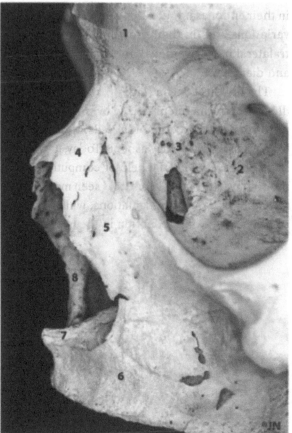

Fig. 41. Lateral view of the skull

1. frontal	6. partially reabsorbed
2. orbit	maxillary
3. lacrimal	alveolar process
4. nasal	7. anterior nasal spine
5. frontal process	8. nasal cavity

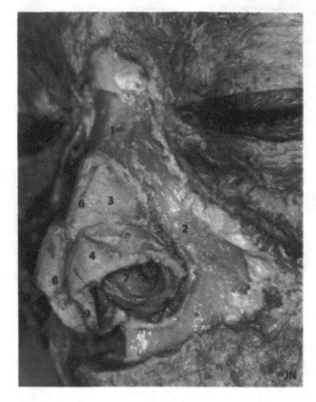

Fig. 42. Anterolateral view of the external nose, left side

1. nasal	6. septum cartilage
2. frontal process	7. nostril
3. superior alar cartilage	8. medial crus
4. inferior alar cartilage	9. lateral crus
5. accessory cartilage	

in their endonasal route. Depending on anatomical variations and on their growth patterns, the contralateral nasal openings can vary widely in shape and diameter.

The bullous concha (Fig. 39), which is the middle nasal concha pneumatized by one or more anterior or posterior ethmoidal cells, was described by Zuckerkandl as early as 1898. Today, it can easily be observed with the help of computerized tomography. The bullous concha is seen mostly in association with septum deviations, which occur to compensate for the reduction in the meatal space.

The compression of the nasal wall of the middle meatus by the bullous concha may result in functional changes in the cellular and sinus drainage through the ostia in the middle meatus, mainly around the ethmoidal bulla and the infundibulum. If the bullous concha is present on both sides and they are volumetrically equivalent, the septum generally does not present any deviation.

Nasal obstructions occurring in the growth phase may interfere with the maxillomandibular complex, altering the dental eruption and the facial morphology.

Chapter 3
Posterior Aperture
of the Nasal Cavity

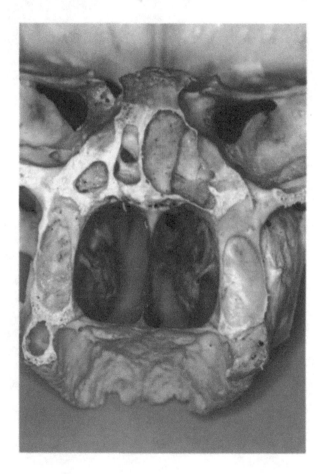

Chapter 3 _____
**Posterior Aperture
of the Nasal Cavity**

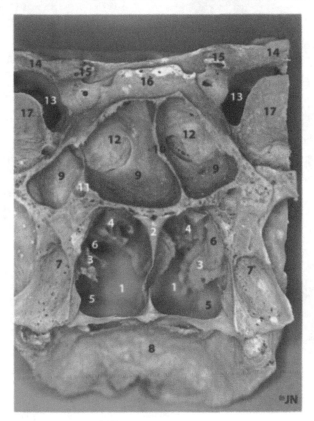

Fig. 43. Bony posterior aperture of nasal cavity

1. choana	11. sphenoidal sinus,
2. nasal septum	accessory septum
3. inferior nasal concha	12. sphenoidal sinus,
4. middle nasal concha	ostium
5. inferior nasal meatus	13. superior orbital fissure
6. middle nasal meatus	14. lesser wing
7. pterygoid process	of the sphenoid
8. palate	15. optic canal
9. sphenoidal sinus	16. hypophysial fossa
10. sphenoidal sinus,	17. greater wing
main septum	of the sphenoid

Through an anteroposterior pyramidal bony tunnel, with the floor of the nasal cavity as a base and the roof as an apex, and the anterior opening narrower than the posterior, we reach the nasopharyngeal transition, termed the posterior opening of the nasal cavity, or choanae, which is divided by the same bony septum as the anterior opening. While the choanae are divided by the vomer, the anterior opening is divided by the septal cartilage (Fig. 43).

The choanal bony boundaries are constituted superiorly by the body of the sphenoid and the wings of the vomer, inferiorly by the palatine horizontal plates, which join in the median suture to form the posterior nasal spine. The medial plates of the pterygoid process of the sphenoid articulate bilaterally with the palatine vertical plates in order to complete the nasopharyngeal border. The choanae are generally oval, with a vertical long axis (Fig. 44).

The superior nasal concha may be seen as a projection extending anteroposteriorly, starting near the nasal roof. It is pneumatized by one or two posterior ethmoidal cells (Onodi cells), filling in most of the superior nasal meatus. The more voluminous these cells, the smaller the meatus, which is located very close to the end of the middle nasal concha, the lower insertion of which favors the expansion of the posterior ethmoidal cells (Fig. 47).

The middle nasal concha varies considerably in size, resembling a narrow, laterally opened „C" that projects towards the nasal septum, almost reaching its bony portion. A large ethmoidal bulla may also occur under the middle nasal concha, reducing the middle nasal meatus even more. Under the meatal prolongation of the middle nasal concha is the dorsum of the usually voluminous inferior nasal concha, which is horizontally disposed, extending to the maxillary nasal wall and to the inferior portions of the ethmoid and lacrimal bones (Figs. 45–48). The inferior and the middle nasal conchae are anatomically very similar, but the former is more frequently hypertrophied due to its valvular arteriovenous structural characteristics, forming a turgescent cavernous system.

Under the inferior nasal concha is a maxillary wall, very concave to the nasal cavity and convex to the maxillary sinus.

The nasal septum may present deviations, exostoses, and spurs, which are more frequently found in its anterior portion (Fig. 44).

Occlusions, perforations, and atrophy of the choanae are generally associated with congenital malformations such as hard palate deformities, fa-

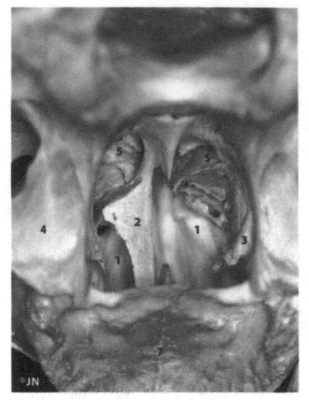

Fig. 44. Bony posterior aperture of nasal cavity, adult

1. choana	4. pterygoid process
2. nasal septum	5. posterior ethmoidal cells
with left deviation	6. foramen magnum
3. inferior nasal concha	7. palate

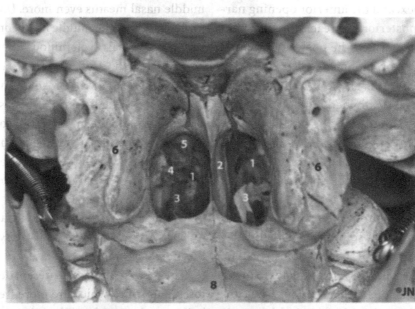

Fig. 45. Bony posterior aperture of nasal cavity, 2-year-old child

1. choana	3. inferior nasal concha	5. middle nasal concha	7. sphenoidal body
2. nasal septum	4. middle nasal meatus	6. pterygoid process	8. palate

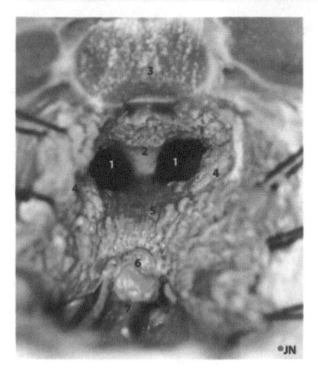

Fig. 46. Bony posterior aperture of nasal cavity, 8-month-old child

1. choana	5. soft palate
2. nasal septum	6. uvula
3. sphenoidal body	7. epiglottis
4. pharynx, lateroposterior wall	

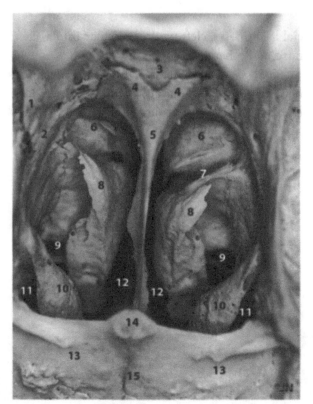

Fig. 47. Bony posterior aperture of nasal cavity, adult

1. medial plate of the pterygoid process	8. middle nasal concha
2. palatine vertical plate	9. middle nasal meatus
3. sphenoidal body	10. inferior nasal concha
4. ala vomer	11. inferior nasal meatus
5. vomer vertical plate	12. common nasal meatus
6. superior nasal concha (pneumatized)	13. palatine horizontal plate
7. superior nasal meatus	14. posterior nasal spine
	15. palate

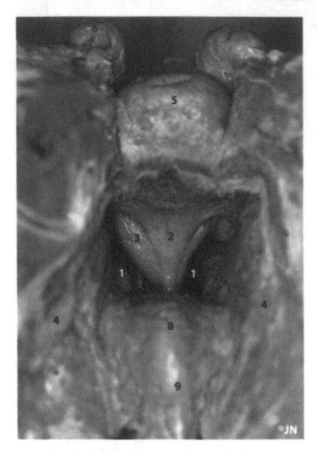

Fig. 48. Posterior aperture of nasal cavity, adult

1. choana	6. left internal carotid artery
2. nasal septum	7. right internal carotid artery
3. adenovascular formation (Almeida)	8. soft palate
4. pharynx, lateral wall	9. uvula
5. left sphenoidal sinus	

cial asymmetry, cleft uvula, auricular fistula, cleft nose, and other pathologies.

Some aspects of the growth of the bony choanae and of the membranous choanae in the cadaver are shown in Figs. 45 and 46.

Figure 48 shows the adenovascular formation near the posterior border of the septum and close to the choanal apertures, as described by Almeida. It can be found either unilaterally or bilaterally.

Chapter 4
Lateral Wall
of the Nasal Cavity

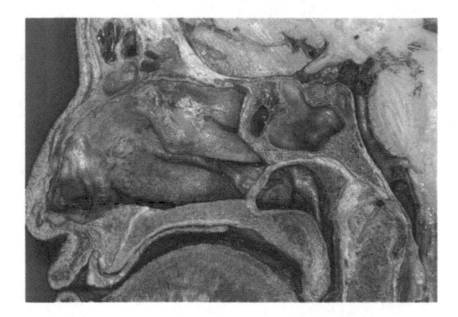

Chapter 4 _____
**Lateral Wall
of the Nasal Cavity**

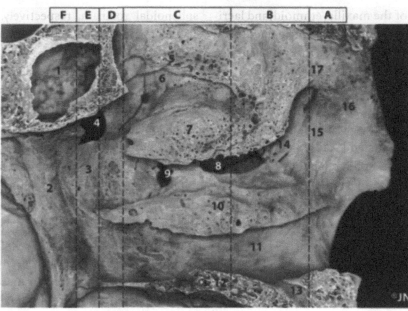

Fig. 49. Bony lateral wall of nasal cavity, left side

1. sphenoidal sinus	5. superior nasal concha	10. inferior nasal concha	15. aditus of middle nasal
2. medial plate	6. superior nasal meatus	11. inferior nasal meatus	meatus
of pterygoid process	7. middle nasal concha	12. palate	16. maxillary frontal process
3. palatine vertical plate	8. anterior window	13. incisive canal	17. agger nasi
4. sphenopalatine foramen	9. posterior window	14. nasolacrimal duct	

Regions, according to thickness of bony wall:

A. maxillary frontal	B. nasolacrimal duct	D. maxillopalatine junction	F. pterygoid process
process	C. middle nasal meatus	E. palatine vertical plate	

The nasal cavity is a quadrangular prism with a larger base as the floor, a smaller base as the roof, and two vertical walls, one lateral and another medial (nasal septum). The lateral walls are both anatomically and functionally more complex than the other walls.

The lateral wall of the nasal cavity is quadrangular and is constituted by parts of the maxilla, ethmoid, lacrimal, nasal, palatine, and sphenoid bones. Its anterior border is constituted by the frontal process of the maxilla and by the nasal bone. It is a compact (Fig. 49, A) and thick region, delimiting a great part of the piriform aperture.

The maxilla has a concave segment in the inferior meatus and in the nasal floor. The inferior nasal concha articulates with the superior border of the inferior meatus. It is usually thin, fusiform, superiorly and medially convex, and inferiorly and laterally concave. In its anterior one third it articulates with the frontal process of the maxilla and the lacrimal bone; in its medial one third it articulates with the uncinate process of the ethmoid, which delimits two openings found in the bony structure of the nasal middle meatus called the anterior and posterior windows, or fontanelles. The fontanelles remain obstructed by the nasal and sinusal mucosae, both in the cadaver and in the living.

The inferior nasal concha has a large anterior head, followed by a large body that converges to form a thin or a thick tail, depending on the degree of mucosal hypertrophy. Under the anterior one third of this concha opens the funnel-shaped nasolacrimal duct. The ethmoidal portion of the lateral wall of the nasal cavity starts above the inferior concha. This is a thin and delicate bony plate, formed by parts of the maxilla, ethmoid, and lacrimal bones. It corresponds to the entire middle nasal meatus under the middle concha, which in turn separates it from the superior nasal meatus.

The middle nasal concha is usually smaller than the inferior one, but it has the same anatomical features. Its head is juxtaposed to the frontal process of the maxilla while its end (tail) is tangent to the inferior edge of the sphenopalatine foramen. A prominence is observed at the point where the head of the middle nasal concha is inserted, corresponding to the region of the agger nasi, with one or two anterior ethmoidal cells distal to the frontal process of the maxilla, lying over the junction of the lacrimal sac with the nasolacrimal duct. Generally, the nasolacrimal duct appears as a small oblique convexity in a superoinferior and anteroposterior position. This is a structure of average thickness (Fig. 49, B). Distal to this area and up to the anterior border of the uncinate process, no bony structure is to be seen, either in the cadaver or in the living, but only nasal and sinusal mucosae obstructing the anterior window of the maxilla. The uncinate process follows as an osseous prolongation of the ethmoid, almost parallel to the nasolacrimal duct. The uncinate process begins at the agger nasi and ends almost imperceptibly near the dorsum of the inferior nasal concha. Next to it is the posterior window, somewhat smaller than the anterior one, also obstructed by mucosa and delimiting this most fragile portion of the lateral wall (Fig. 49, C). At the level of the end (tail) of the inferior and middle nasal conchae is a resistant osseous pillar – the maxillopalatine junction – (Fig. 49, D), bordering the pterygopalatine fossa anteromedially. Following the maxillopalatine junction is the vertical plate of the palatine bone (Fig. 49, E). This is a rather thin laminar structure, with dehiscences through which the palatine vasculonervous pedicles reach the nasal cavity. It also constitutes the medial wall of the pterygopalatine fossa, with the sphenopalatine foramen opening in its superior end. The sphenopalatine foramen is bordered by the orbital and sphenoidal processes of the palatine bone, which articulate with the ethmoid and the

sphenoidal rostrum, respectively. The last bony segment of the lateral wall is constituted by the medial plate of the pterygoid process of the sphenoid (Fig. 49, F). It is a region as thick as the frontal process of the maxilla and constitutes the lateral border of the choana. The middle nasal concha is very important, due to the site where it inserts in the lateral wall of the nasal cavity, representing the basal lamella of the embryonic stage, which delimits the anterior (anteroinferior) and posterior (posterosuperior) triangles where the ethmoidal cells take their origin and keep their drainage ostia. Thus, the ethmoidal cells are split into two groups – the anterior and the posterior. This classification is consequently also valid for the paranasal sinuses, since they originate from the ethmoidal cells. The basal lamella, like the concha itself, is superoinferiorly and anteroposteriorly oblique in relation to the lateral wall of the nasal cavity and the orbital wall of the ethmoid (lamina papyracea).

Above the middle nasal concha is the superior nasal meatus, much smaller than the middle meatus. It is bordered anteriorly by the superior and middle conchae and posteriorly by the sphenoidal recess. In this small space, frequently filled by posterior ethmoidal cells, the same anatomical elements can be seen as in the middle meatus, such as the ethmoidal bulla, semilunar hiatus, infundibulum, and uncinate process, although very reduced in size. Distal to the superior nasal concha, a small space may be present in 48% of cases (Lang) – the sphenoethmoidal recess, where the ostium of the sphenoidal sinus is found. A fourth nasal concha, described by Zuckerkandl as the „concha suprema", may be present as a reduced, often pneumatized process. Figure 50 shows the right lateral wall of the nasal cavity, from which the meatal prolongation of the middle nasal concha has been removed, leaving its dorsum and base of insertion (basal lamella) in the nasal bony wall.

Observe that the head of the middle nasal concha is inserted very close to the roof of the nasal cavity, beside the cribriform plate of the ethmoid. It descends backwards in an oblique route until it ends under the sphenopalatine foramen. If this

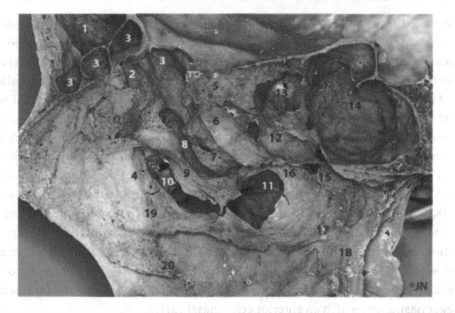

Fig. 50. Bony lateral wall of nasal cavity, right side

1. frontal sinus	6. middle nasal concha	12. superior nasal meatus	17. palatine vertical plate
2. agger nasi	7. ethmoidal bulla	13. posterior ethmoidal cell	18. medial plate
3. anterior ethmoidal cell	8. semilunar hiatus	14. sphenoidal sinus	of pterygoid process
4. aditus of middle nasal	9. uncinate process	15. sphenopalatine foramen	19. inferior nasal concha
meatus	10. anterior fontanelle	16. tail of middle nasal	20. inferior nasal meatus
5. small portion	11. posterior fontanelle	concha	
of the nasal septum			

foramen is double or multiple, the bony end (tail) of the middle concha ends between the largest (superior) and the lesser (inferior) one. As explained before, the basal lamella divides the ethmoidal cells into an anterior and a posterior group. Some ethmoidal cells are found anterosuperiorly under the ethmoidal recess, lateral to the cribriform plate of the ethmoid. The most anterior cells near the frontonasal recess extend over the area of the lacrimal sac and the most superior portion of the lacrimal duct, which is located between this group of cells and the uncinate process of the ethmoid, as a small projection situated similar to the middle nasal concha (Fig. 50).

The uncinate process is a secondary nasal concha with an inverted position, whose head would be at the region of the agger nasi. Its line of insertion and nasal prolongation delimit the infundibulum, a groove in a similar disposition originating in a blind end in the frontoethmoidal recess, where the ethmoidal cells and/or the ostium of the frontal sinus open. Above the semilunar hiatus is a regular, curved, and superiorly concave space – the semilunar hiatus – and right above it is the ethmoidal bulla, usually constituted by an anterior ethmoidal cell. The ethmoidal bulla grows beneath the middle nasal concha and, depending on the degree of pneumatization, may display a most variable anatomy, being generally inferiorly convex and superiorly concave. It occasionally resembles an uncinate process with little pneumatization. The space or recess seen above the ethmoidal bulla is the lateral sinus, or suprabullar recess, where the anterior ethmoidal cells and the ethmoidal bulla open.

The ethmoidal bulla is regarded as an important ethmoidal cell owing to its strategic position, serving as a base for the nasal ethmoid, while the uncinate process is located in the transition between the maxillary and the ethmoidal sinuses. The ethmoidal bulla can grow so as to reach superiorly the ethmoidal fovea and the lateral side of the cribriform lamina of the ethmoid.

In a normal nasal cavity, all the structures of the lateral wall are in harmonious proportions (Fig. 51–53). Anterior to the nasal aditus, at the transition between the vestibule and the nasal cavity, the nasal limen is seen as a valvular constriction representing the threshold from the external nose to the nasal cavity. The smooth and regular region that follows is the frontal process of the maxilla, which articulates with the nasal bone up to the nasofrontal articulation. Somewhat below and distal is the aditus of the middle nasal meatus, where the head of the middle nasal concha is located. A prominence in this superior area is the agger nasi, above which an anterior cell is shown without its nasal wall. The nasal septum reflected upwards prevents a view of the nasal roof. All this wide superior region ends posteriorly in the small superior nasal concha and in the narrow and long middle nasal concha. Both conchae end at the anterior wall of the sphenoidal si-nus, anterior to the sphenoethmoidal recess. The superior nasal meatus is elongated and narrow, with a cellular ostium near its end (tail). The middle nasal concha is fusiform and also elongated, with its tail under the sphenoidal rostrum. The region of the sphenopalatine foramen communicates the pterygopalatine fossa with the nasal cavity. In the skull, the sphenopalatine foramen is above the tail of the middle nasal concha, but in the cadaver and in the living, due to the variable thickness of the nasal lining, it may be seen in close relationship with the posterior one fourth of the tail. This area should be manipulated with caution because of the presence of vasculonervous pedicles traversing the foramen towards the nasal cavity.

The inferior nasal concha is voluminous and regular in shape, presenting a head and a tail of variable thickness, depending on turgescence. Longitudinal stretches are occasionally seen on the dorsum of the inferior nasal concha, enlarging the area of nasal mucosa in it. The inferior

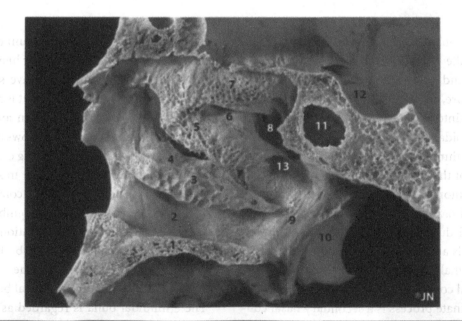

Fig. 51. Bony lateral wall of nasal cavity, right side

1. palate	5. middle nasal concha	8. sphenoethmoidal recess	11. sphenoidal sinus
2. inferior nasal meatus	6. superior nasal meatus	9. nasochoanal region	12. hypophysial fossa
3. inferior nasal concha	7. superior nasal concha	10. pterygoid process	13. sphenopalatine foramen
4. middle nasal meatus			

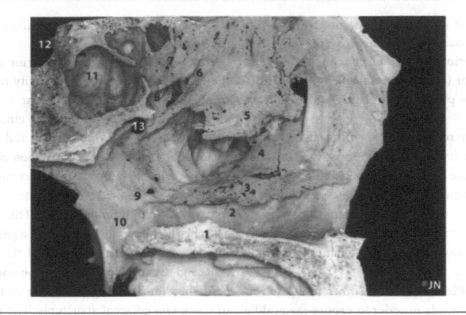

Fig. 52. Bony lateral wall of nasal cavity, left side

1. palate	5. middle nasal concha	8. sphenoethmoidal recess	11. sphenoidal sinus
2. inferior nasal meatus	6. superior nasal meatus	9. nasochoanal region	12. hypophysial fossa
3. inferior nasal concha	7. superior nasal concha	10. pterygoid process	13. sphenopalatine foramen
4. middle nasal meatus			

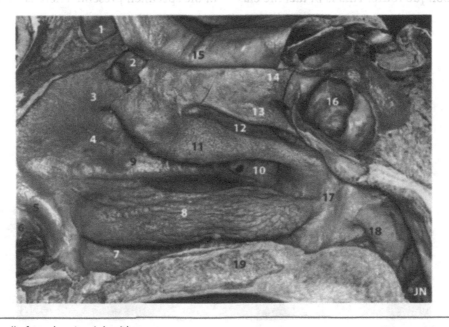

Fig. 53. Lateral wall of nasal cavity, right side

1. frontal sinus	6. nostril	11. middle nasal concha	17. choanal region
2. anterior ethmoidal cell	7. inferior nasal meatus	12. superior nasal meatus	18. pharyngeal aperture
3. agger nasi	8. inferior nasal concha	13. superior nasal concha	of auditory tube
4. aditus of middle nasal	9. middle nasal meatus	14. supreme nasal concha	19. palate
meatus	10. accessory ostium	15. nasal septum (reflected)	
5. nasal limen	of maxillary sinus	16. sphenoidal sinus	

nasal meatus in the specimen shown in the figures here is narrow and concave to the nasal cavity; the inferior and middle conchae converge to the posterior (choanal) nasal space, and just behind it is the pharyngeal opening of the auditory tube.

The numerous structures of the lateral wall of the nasal cavity may display a most varied anatomy within the limits of normality (Fig. 54–68). It should be kept in mind that these structures are extremely dynamic in the living, possessing secretory functions, besides being permanently subject to environmental oscillations, trauma, and diseases.

The middle nasal concha shown in Fig. 58 was deflected upwards in order to expose the middle nasal meatus and its anatomical elements. Note that the insertion of the middle nasal concha is not as horizontal as it appears in the skull; rather, it starts in the most anterior, superior, and lateral portion, close to the nasal roof, descending posteriorly in an oblique route. This is in fact the clas-

sical disposition of the basal lamella of the middle nasal concha.

In the most anterior and superior portions of the middle nasal meatus a concavity leads to the frontoethmoidal recess. Somewhat behind is a small prominence of an anterior ethmoidal cell from the nasal bony region. Below and anterior to the middle nasal concha is the region of the agger nasi. The uncinate process starts there as a thin tail distal to the ethmoidal bulla, resembling a regular fold with a location similar to that of the middle nasal concha. The semilunar hiatus is a gap intervening between the inferior border of the ethmoidal bulla and the superior border of the uncinate process. The width of this gap depends on the volume of those two adjacent structures. The infundibulum, seen as a canal at the bottom of the hiatus, is determined by the insertion of the uncinate process in the nasal lateral wall. Furthermore, it may contain several cellular ostia and the openings of the maxillary and frontal sinuses. The ethmoidal bulla in the specimen presented here is superiorly regu-

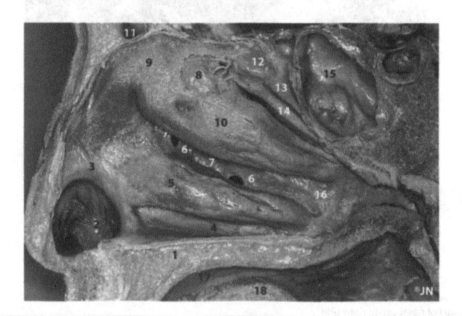

Fig. 54. Lateral wall of nasal cavity, right side

1. palate	6. accessory ostium	10. middle nasal concha	15. sphenoidal sinus
2. nostril	of maxillary sinus	11. frontal sinus	16. choanal region
3. nasal limen	7. middle nasal meatus	12. posterior ethmoidal cell	17. oral cavity
4. inferior nasal meatus	8. anterior ethmoidal cell	13. supreme nasal concha	18. tongue
5. inferior nasal concha	9. agger nasi	14. superior nasal concha	

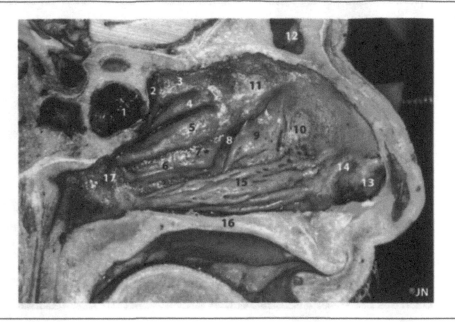

Fig. 55. Lateral wall of nasal cavity, left side

1. sphenoidal sinus	5. middle nasal concha	10. middle meatus aditus	15. middle nasal concha
2. sphenoethmoidal	6. middle nasal meatus	11. agger nasi	16. palate
recess	7. ethmoidal bulla	12. frontal sinus	17. choanal region
3. supreme nasal concha	8. semilunar hiatus	13. nostril	
4. superior nasal concha	9. uncinate process	14. nasal limen	

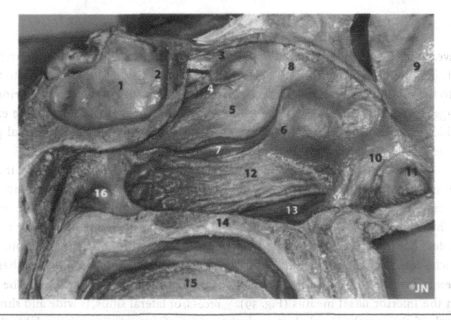

Fig. 56. Lateral wall of nasal cavity, left side

1. main septum	4. superior nasal meatus	9. nasal septum (reflected)	14. palate
of sphenoidal sinus	5. middle nasal concha	10. nasal limen	15. tongue
2. ostium of sphenoidal	6. uncinate process	11. nostril	16. pharyngeal aperture
sinus (red probe)	7. middle nasal meatus	12. inferior nasal concha	of auditory tube
3. superior nasal concha	8. agger nasi	13. inferior nasal meatus	

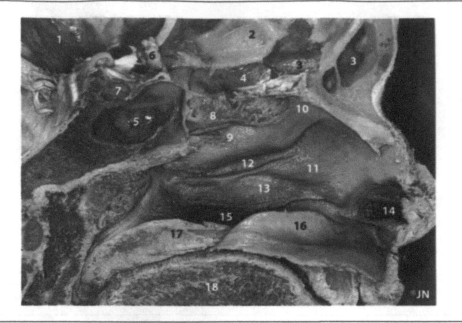

Fig. 57. Lateral wall of nasal cavity, left side

1. medial cranial fossa	7. hypophysis	12. middle nasal meatus	16. septum of nasal cavity,
2. anterior cranial fossa	8. superior nasal concha	13. inferior nasal concha,	with left deviation,
3. frontal sinus	9. middle nasal concha	depressed by the	resected and reflected
4. anterior ethmoidal cell	10. agger nasi	nasal septum	to the right
5. sphenoidal sinus	11. aditus of middle	14. nostril	17. palate
6. optic nerve	nasal meatus	15. inferior nasal meatus	18. tongue

lar and concave, giving origin to the suprabullar recess or lateral sinus, where the anterior cells open.

Anterior to the middle nasal meatus, the nasal walls of the agger nasi are exposed by the deflection of the middle nasal concha (Fig. 59). The most posterior of these cells can be seen to expand toward the uncinate process, pneumatizing it. The great proximity commonly observed between the uncinate process and the nasolacrimal duct does not occur in this case. The bony nasal wall of the nasolacrimal duct has been removed and the inferior nasal concha resected in its anterior one third to afford a view to the draining site of the nasolacrimal duct in the inferior nasal meatus (Fig. 59). The nasal wall of the nasolacrimal duct varies greatly in thickness and degree of prominence.

The proximity of the maxillary sinus to the nasolacrimal duct has long been observed by authors such as Sieur and Jacob, Zuckerkandl, Killian, and more recently Skillern and others. This an-

atomical relationship should be considered in surgical cases where endonasal access to the nasolacrimal duct is sought, since the lacrimal recess of the maxillary sinus is, to a variable extent, interposed between the maxillary frontal process and the nasolacrimal duct.

In the specimen presented here, the pneumatization of the uncinate process does not cause a narrowing of the semilunar hiatus. The infundibulum appears more obvious because the uncinate process is inserted in a higher position. An anterior ethmoidal cell, whose nasal wall has been removed, is seen at the anterobullar space. The suprabullar recess, or lateral sinus, is wide and shows the large ostium of an anterior ethmoidal cell. Under the bulla and distal to the uncinate process, the wall of the middle nasal meatus is regular and presents a relatively large accessory ostium for the maxillary sinus in a central position. The inferior nasal concha, although resected, shows longitudinal stretch-

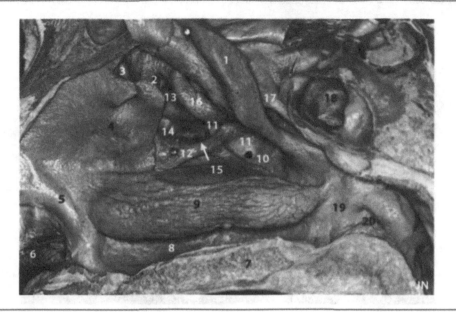

Fig. 58. Lateral wall of nasal cavity, right side

1. middle nasal concha (reflected)	6. nostril	12. uncinate process	17. superior nasal concha
2. frontoethmoidal recess	7. palate	13. semilunar hiatus	18. sphenoidal sinus
3. agger nasi	8. inferior nasal meatus	14. infundibular canal	19. choanal region
4. aditus of middle meatus	9. inferior nasal concha	15. main ostium of maxillary sinus (arrow)	20. pharyngeal aperture of auditory tube
5. nasal limen	10. middle nasal meatus	16. ethmoidal bulla	
	11. accessory ostium of maxillary sinus		

es. Its thin tail favors a wide transition from the middle nasal meatus to the choanal region.

The superior nasal meatus is usually small and without very differentiated anatomical structures. The deflection of the superior nasal concha by a vertical incision shows the anterosuperior recess, where posterior ethmoidal cells open, followed by an indistinctly visible ethmoidal bulla (Fig. 66). Under the bulla, a wide recess continues posteriorly to the sphenoethmoidal recess. The supreme nasal concha and the superior nasal concha share a small area located posterosuperiorly in the lateral wall of the nasal cavity. However, if the superior nasal meatus is wide, the supreme concha is nonexistent. If the most posterior ethmoidal cells are excessively voluminous, the whole region becomes pneumatized, the sphenoethmoidal recess disappears, and the ostium of the sphenoid sinus moves closer to the nasal septum, maintaining, however, the vertical distance to the nasal roof of about 8 mm. The posterior ethmoi-

dal cells are more cranial than the anterior cells and the cribriform lamina, extending from distal to the crista galli and the cribriform lamina of the ethmoid to the lesser wing of the sphenoid.

The mucosal lining of the conchae and superior meatus is mostly olfactory, being supplied by ethmoidal ophthalmic branches.

The superior meatus and the superior nasal conchae are very close to one another. Therefore, the posterior ethmoidal cells and the ethmoidal sinus share a common draining route towards the nasopharynx.

The sectioning of the anterior one third of the middle nasal concha exposes part of the agger nasi cell and of an ethmoidal suprabullar cell. The middle nasal concha is apparently pneumatized by a cell which is, in fact, a bullar concha extending towards the superior nasal meatus (Fig. 67). The cells invading this concha vary in number from one to three, according to Sieur and Jacob. Since the pneu-

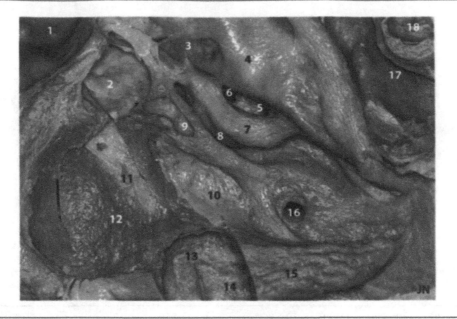

Fig. 59. Lateral wall of nasal cavity, right side

1. frontal sinus	6. ostium of anterior ethmoidal cell	11. nasolacrimal duct, nasal wall	14. inferior nasal meatus
2. agger nasi	7. ethmoidal bulla	12. aditus of middle nasal meatus	15. inferior nasal concha (resected)
3. anterior ethmoidal cell	8. semilunar hiatus	13. region of the nasolacrimal duct's nasal aperture	16. accessory ostium of maxillary sinus
4. middle nasal concha (reflected)	9. uncinate process (pneumatized)		17. sphenoethmoidal recess
5. lateral sinus	10. middle nasal meatus		18. sphenoidal sinus

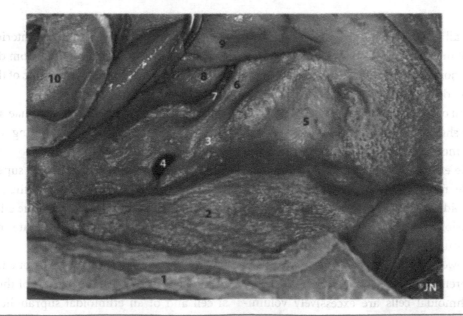

Fig. 60. Left lateral wall of nasal cavity

1. palate	4. accessory ostium of maxillary sinus	6. uncinate process	9. middle nasal concha
2. inferior nasal concha	5. aditus of middle nasal meatus	7. semilunar hiatus	10. septum of sphenoidal sinus
3. middle nasal meatus		8. ethmoidal bulla	

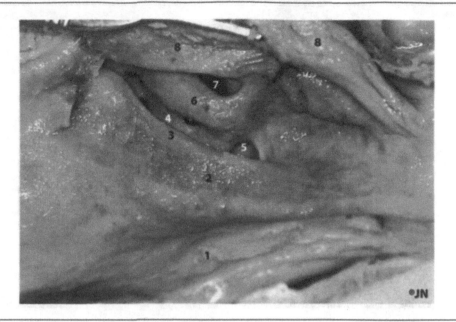

Fig. 61. Right lateral wall of nasal cavity

1. inferior nasal concha	4. semilunar hiatus	6. ethmoidal bulla	8. middle nasal concha
2. middle nasal meatus	5. accessory ostium	7. lateral sinus	(reflected)
3. uncinate process	of maxillary sinus		

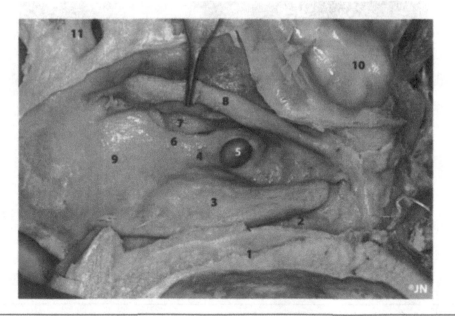

Fig. 62. Right lateral wall of nasal cavity

1. palate	4. middle nasal meatus	7. ethmoidal bulla	9. aditus of middle
2. inferior nasal meatus	5. accessory ostium	8. middle nasal concha	nasal meatus
3. inferior nasal concha	of maxillary sinus	(reflected)	10. sphenoidal sinus
	6. uncinate process		11. frontal sinus

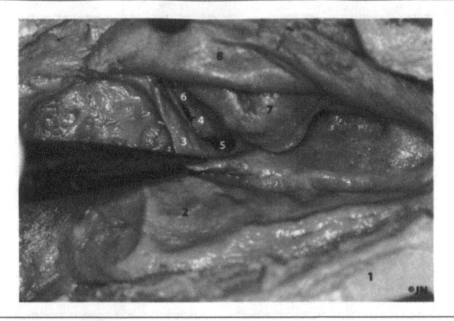

Fig. 63. Right lateral wall of nasal cavity

1. palate	3. uncinate process	5. main ostium	7. ethmoidal bulla
2. inferior nasal concha	(reflected)	of maxillary sinus	8. middle nasal concha
	4. semilunar hiatus	6. infundibulum	(reflected)

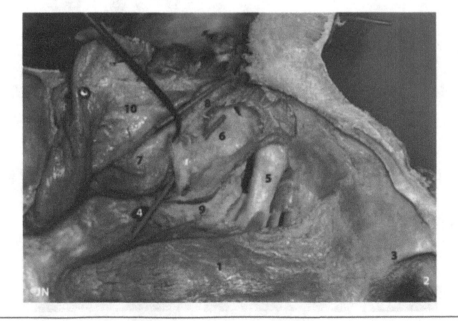

Fig. 64. Left lateral wall of nasal cavity

1. inferior nasal concha	5. nasolacrimal duct without	7. ethmoidal bulla	9. middle nasal meatus
2. nostril	the bony nasal wall	8. the probe emerges	10. middle nasal concha
3. nasal limen	6. pneumatized uncinate	from the frontal sinus,	(reflected)
4. accessory ostium	process with probe	in the region	
of maxillary sinus	in its interior	of the nasofrontal recess	

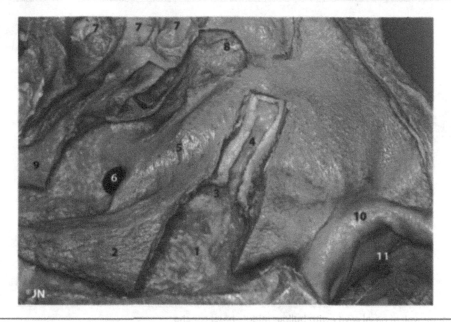

Fig. 65. Left lateral wall of nasal cavity

1. inferior nasal meatus	4. nasolacrimal duct	7. ethmoidal cells	10. nasal limen
2. inferior nasal concha	with nasal wall removed	without nasal walls	11. nostril
(resected)	5. middle nasal meatus	8. agger nasi	
3. nasolacrimal duct	6. accessory ostium	9. middle nasal concha	
aperture	of maxillary sinus	(resected)	

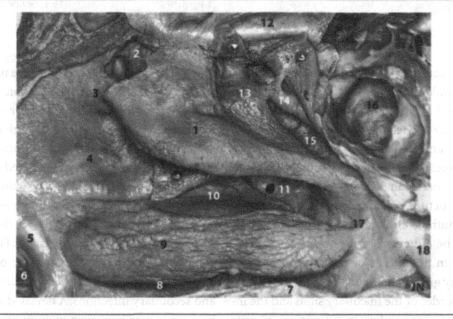

Fig. 66. Right lateral wall of nasal cavity

1. middle nasal concha	7. palate	12. superior nasal concha	15. sphenoethmoidal
2. frontoethmoidal recess	8. inferior nasal meatus	(reflected)	recess
3. agger nasi	9. inferior nasal concha	13. superior nasal meatus	16. sphenoidal sinus
4. aditus of middle meatus	10. middle nasal meatus	14. recess with ostia	17. choanal region
5. nasal limen	11. accessory ostium	of posterior	18. pharyngeal aperture
6. nostril	of maxillary sinus	ethmoidal cells	of auditory tube

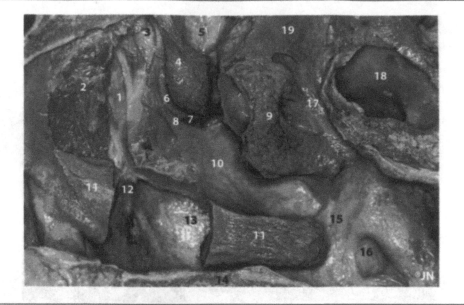

Fig. 67. Right lateral wall of nasal cavity with bullous middle nasal concha

1. nasolacrimal duct	7. main ostium	11. inferior nasal concha	15. choanal region
2. frontal process	of maxillary sinus	(resected)	16. pharyngeal aperture
3. agger nasi cell	8. uncinate process	12. nasal aperture	of auditory tube
4. ethmoidal bulla	9. middle bullous	of nasolacrimal duct	17. sphenoethmoidal
5. suprabullar ethmoidal cell	nasal concha	(*with probe*)	recess
6. semilunar hiatus	10. middle nasal meatus	13. inferior nasal meatus	18. sphenoidal sinus
		14. palate	19. superior nasal concha

matization occurs at the level of the basal lamella, these cells could have their origin in the middle or superior nasal meatus, as reported by Hajek.

The bullar concha was first described by Zuckerkandl and Killian over a century ago. In fact, the bullar concha and the maxillo-orbital cells (Haller cells) have occasionally been referred to as being the same structure, causing some misunderstanding among authors and readers. The maxillo-orbital cells can be either posterior or anterior, having their origin in the middle or in the superior nasal meatus. They grow in the space between the posterosuperior border of the maxillary sinus and the infraorbital space, expanding in a direction opposite the bullar concha, i.e., towards the infraorbital space. If the pneumatization of the middle nasal concha is more anterior, it is probably an anterior ethmoidal cell. If more than one cell is present, they could have a double origin. The ostia of the conchal cells are frequently near the concave nasal wall, under the concha, close to its insertion in the suprabullar space. The presence of such pneumatizations has aroused growing interest through the years, due to their clinical and surgical implications. Their occurrence, either isolated or associated with a hypertrophy of the ethmoidal bulla or with a pneumatization of the uncinate process and with septal deviations, may significantly reduce the functional respiratory space of the nasal cavity. Further, such a condition may impair the drainage of the sinuses and ethmoidal cells, leading to mucous retention and secondary infections. A deviated septum could be a consequence of such pneumatization, but it is also genetically determined, since it is already observed in the fetal stage. Today, thanks to computerized tomography (Figs. 69, 70), the bullar concha is more easily identified, being detected in as many as 50% of individuals.

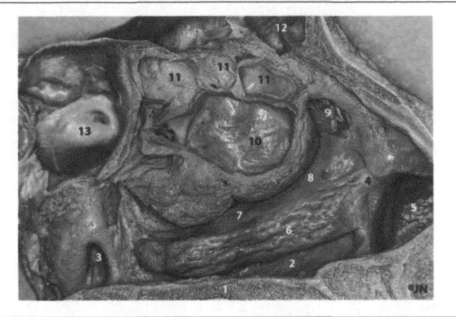

Fig. 68. Left lateral wall of nasal cavity with large middle bullous nasal concha

1. palate	4. nasal limen	8. aditus of middle	11. ethmoidal cells
2. inferior nasal meatus	5. nostril	nasal meatus	12. frontal sinus
3. pharyngeal opening	6. inferior nasal concha	9. agger nasi cell	13. sphenoidal sinus
of auditory tube	7. middle nasal meatus	10. middle bullous	
		nasal concha	

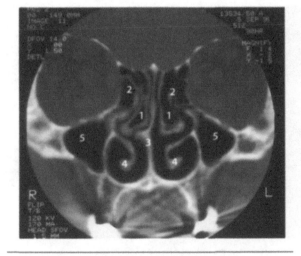

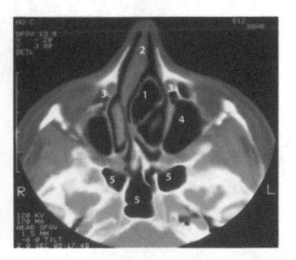

Fig. 69. Coronal CT of nasal cavity and paranasal sinuses

1. middle bullous	3. nasal septum with
nasal concha (bilateral)	deviation to the right
2. ethmoidal bulla	4. inferior nasal concha
	5. maxillary sinus

(Reproduced with thanks to Dr. Rainer Haetinger, Med Imagem, São Paulo, Brazil)

Fig. 70. Axial CT of nasal cavity and paranasal sinuses

1. middle bullous	3. nasolacrimal duct
nasal concha (left side)	4. maxillary sinus
2. nasal septum with	5. sphenoidal sinus
deviation to the right	

(Reproduced with thanks to Dr. Rainer Haetinger, Med Imagem, São Paulo, Brazil)

Chapter 5
Nasal Septum

Chapter 5
Nasal Septum

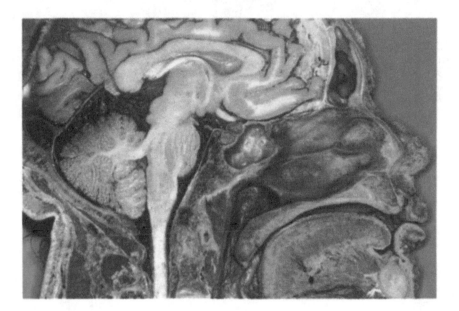

Chapter 5 _____
Nasal Septum

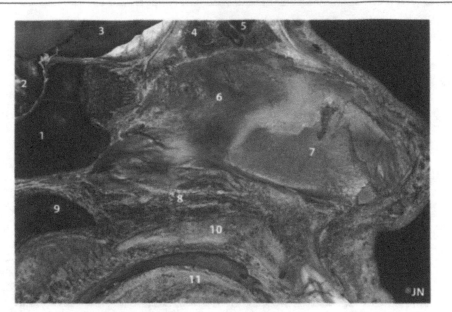

Fig. 71. Nasal septum, right side

1. main septum of sphenoidal sinus	3. anterior cranial fossa	6. ethmoidal perpendicular plate	9. choanal region
2. hypophysis	4. crista galli	7. nasal septum cartilage	10. palate
	5. frontal sinus	8. vomer	11. tongue

The nasal septum divides the nasal cavity into two parts, the right and the left, from the nostrils to the choanae. It is an osteocartilaginous structure, with membranous insertions binding the cartilage to the bony skeleton.

The bony portion of the nasal septum is constituted superoanteriorly by the perpendicular plate of the ethmoid and superoposteriorly and inferiorly by the vomer. These two sagittal bony plates articulate diagonally, forming an anterior concave edge, usually in the sagittal plane. The somewhat quadrilateral cartilaginous portion of the nasal septum, known as the nasal septum cartilage, articulates with this concavity. This cartilage may extend toward the sphenoidal sinus, between the ethmoid and the vomer, preventing the fusion of these two bones. Zuckerkandl describes it as the sphenoidal prolongation of the septal cartilage. The septum continues superiorly at the level of the crista galli, in the anterior cranial fossa, constituting the vertical portion of the ethmoid. This process is surrounded by the cribriform lamina like a horse-shoe. The septum is bordered posterosuperiorly by the lesser wing and the body of the sphenoid, following along the free border of the vomer, at the choanae. Anteriorly, it is continuous with the septal cartilage, under the nasal portion of the frontal bone and the nasal bones. These anatomical relationships vary according to genetic factors, race, sex, and growth process, and are also affected by traumas and diseases. Deviations and exostoses are observed as early as during the fetal stage, at the articular and the free areas of the septum. The nasal septum and the main septum of the sphenoidal sinus are frequently seen in the same sagittal plane. The suture lines of the septal elements are well visible even when covered by perichondrium, periosteum, and nasal mucosa. The mucosal lining of the nasal septum is less turgescent than that of the nasal conchae, but more turgescent than the meatal and intrasinusal mucosae (Figs. 71, 72).

The transition septum–roof–lateral wall of the nasal cavity is a narrow and angled space, where olfactory, trigeminal, and vascular ends merge into a

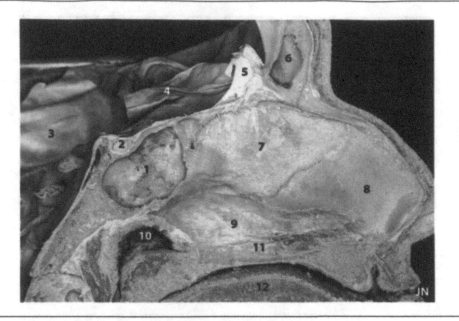

Fig. 72. Nasal septum, right side

1. main septum of sphenoidal sinus	3. middle cranial fossa	7. ethmoidal perpendicular plate	9. vomer
2. hypophysis	4. anterior cranial fossa	8. nasal septum cartilage	10. choanal region
	5. crista galli		11. palate
	6. frontal sinus		12. tongue

special and turgescent mucosa termed the olfactory or pituitary mucosa. At the level of the vomero-cartilaginous junction, near the nasal floor, the mucosa of the nasal septum is turgescent and vascularized by an arteriovenous plexus, as described by Zuckerkandl (Figs. 73–75).

The nasopalatine arteries and nerves descend along the ethmoido-vomerian junction, coming from the sphenoidal portion of the septum to the nasal openings of the incisive canal.

The ethmoidal vasculonervous branches of the ophthalmic artery and nerve descend from the roof and follow together with the arterial and nervous maxillary branches. These vessels and nerves will meet the terminals of the facial artery and facial nerve in the most anterior part of the nasal cavity.

Lymphatic and glandular concentrations have also been described in the anteroposterior regions of the nasal septum, in its nasopharyngeal transition.

Chronic respiratory obstructions occurring in the growth phase may lead to oral breathing, thereby impairing the normal development of the maxillo-mandibular complex.

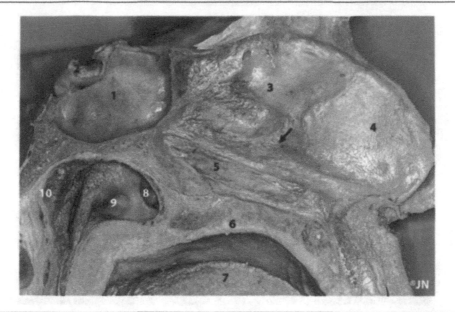

Fig. 73. Nasal septum, right side

1. main septum of sphenoidal sinus 2. hypophysis	3. ethmoid perpendicular plate 4. nasal septum cartilage	5. vomer, with exostoses in its superior border (*arrow*) 6. palate 7. tongue	8. choanal region 9. pharyngeal aperture of auditory tube 10. nasopharynx

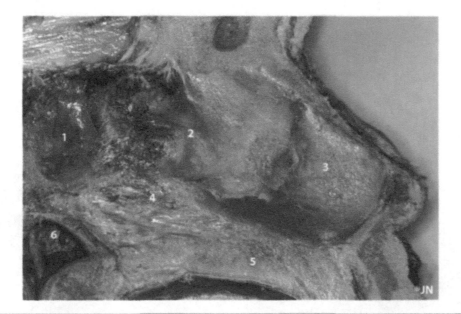

Fig. 74. Nasal septum, right side

1. main septum of sphenoidal sinus	2. ethmoid perpendicular plate	3. nasal septum cartilage 4. vomer	5. palate 6. choanal region

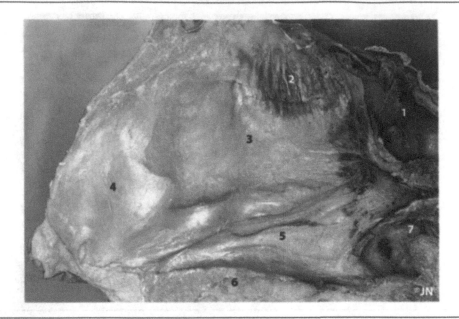

Fig. 75. Nasal septum, left side

1. sphenoidal sinus 2. olfactory region	3. ethmoid perpendicular plate	4. nasal septum cartilage, with sphenoidal enlargement (Zuckerkandl)	5. vomer 6. palate 7. choanal region

Chapter 6
Arteries and Nerves of the Nasal Cavity and Paranasal Sinuses

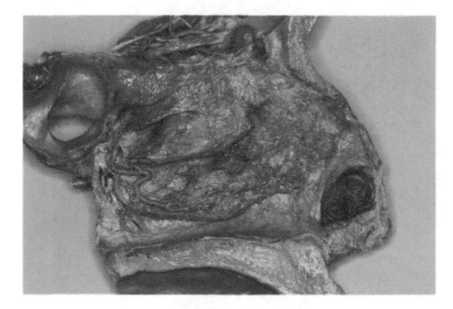

Chapter 6
**Arteries and Nerves
of the Nasal Cavity
and Paranasal Sinuses**

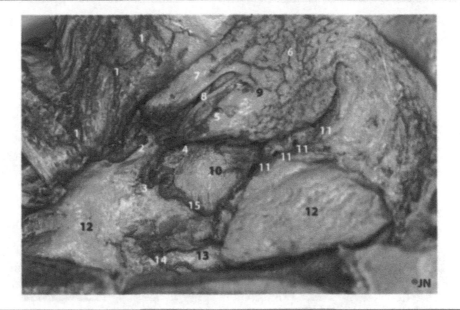

Fig. 76. Lateral wall of nasal cavity and reflected nasal septum, left side

1. septal artery branches 2. septal artery 3. posterior lateral nasal artery 4. middle nasal concha artery	5. arteries to the superior nasal meatus and superior nasal concha 6. anastomosis of the ethmoidal arteries' branches and posterior lateral nasal artery 7. superior nasal concha	8. ostium of posterior ethmoidal cell 9. middle nasal concha 10. middle nasal meatus 11. accessory ostia of maxillary sinus	12. inferior nasal concha (resected) 13. inferior nasal meatus 14. arterial branches of inferior nasal meatus 15. inferior nasal concha artery

The nasal cavity is basically supplied by branches of the maxillary artery and nerve, which derive from the external carotid artery and trigeminal nerve, complemented by branches of the ophthalmic artery and nerves and by branches of the internal carotid artery and trigeminal nerve, respectively.

The maxillary artery pursues a lateromedial route within the pterygopalatine fossa, juxtaposed to the anterior surface of the pterygopalatine ganglion, to which it is attached, being related to several ganglionic nervous ends. In its short length, the maxillary artery emits branches towards the round and palatine canals and the orbit. Still inside the fossa, a few millimeters from the sphenopalatine foramen and towards the nasal cavity, the maxillary artery branches off to give origin to its terminal branches – the septal artery and the posterior lateral nasal artery – which, after a short course, cross the sphenopalatine foramen at its superior and inferior edges, respectively, thus reaching the lateral wall of the nasal cavity (Figs. 76–80). Thin branches may also derive from these two arteries, following the pterygoidal and pterygopalatine canals, besides the lesser palatine branches supplying the hard and soft palate, and others reaching the orbit through the inferior orbital fissure. The septal artery surrounds the superior edge of the sphenopalatine foramen in its course towards the nose, ascending towards the anterior wall of the sphenoidal sinus, where it emits branches to supply all sinusal walls. The branches of the septal artery extend also to the homolateral posterior cells, eventually anastomosing with the contralateral cells at the median sagittal plane (see Fig. 73).

On reaching the nasal septum, the septal artery branches off and spreads out subperiosteally and

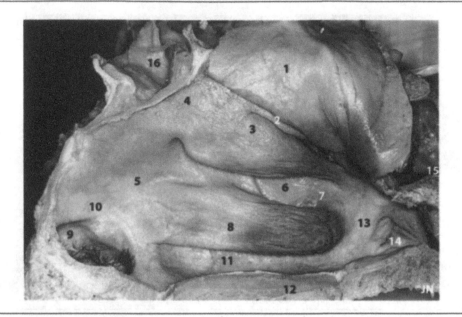

Fig. 77. Right lateral wall of nasal cavity

1. nasal septum (reflected)	6. middle nasal meatus	8. inferior nasal concha	14. pharyngeal aperture
2. superior nasal meatus	7. posterior lateral nasal	9. nostril	of auditory tube
3. middle nasal concha	artery, seen by	10. nasal limen	15. sphenoidal sinus
4. agger nasi	transparency, under	11. inferior nasal meatus	16. frontal sinus
5. aditus of middle nasal	the nasal mucosa	12. palate	
meatus		13. choanal region	

subperichondrially. The nasopalatine artery, one of its largest branches, descends through the vomero-ethmoidal junction together with its nervous homonyms. It reaches the nasal openings of the incisive canal, through which it passes and forms an anastomosis with the contralateral artery to become the incisive artery, which in turn will supply the anterior palate and periosteum. Some branches of the septal artery reach the nasal floor and anastomose with the transosseous branches of the palate; other branches reach the external nose, where they meet branches of the infraorbital and facial arteries. Close to the nasal roof, the ascending branches of the septal artery meet the posterior and anterior branches of the ethmoidal arteries, constituting an important ethmoidoseptal plexus. This plexus, under certain conditions, may be the origin of severe epistaxis. The posterior lateral nasal artery crosses the inferior edge of the sphenopalatine foramen and descends subperiosteally along the lateral wall of the nasal cavity. Some small ascending

branches emerge from the posterior lateral nasal artery as it leaves the sphenopalatine foramen. These branches will supply the superior nasal meatus and the superior nasal concha. At the level of the superior nasal meatus, branches of the posterior lateral nasal artery anastomose with branches of the posterior ethmoidal artery, the same thing occurring in the nasal septum with the septal ends. Near the sphenopalatine foramen, the posterior lateral nasal artery gives off a large-caliber branch to the middle nasal concha that runs periosteally under it and supplies the whole concha, extending to the middle and superior nasal meatus. Next, it descends either vertically or obliquely, in a straight or a tortuous route along the middle meatus, emitting several meatal branches in its course. The posterior lateral nasal artery may be double – in this case, one of them is larger and can easily be distinguished. Branches of this artery to the nasopharyngeal region and tubal opening are also observed. It reaches the inferior nasal concha, spread-

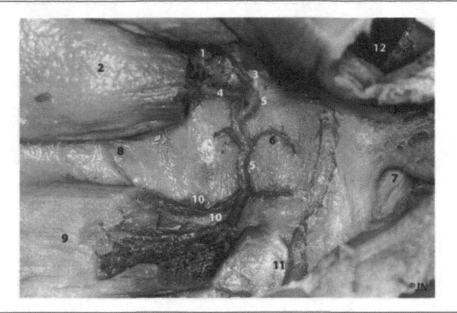

Fig. 78. Right lateral wall of nasal cavity

1. superior nasal meatus	4. middle nasal concha artery	7. pharyngeal aperture of auditory tube	10. inferior nasal concha artery
2. middle nasal concha (resected)	5. posterior lateral nasal artery	8. middle nasal meatus	11. arteries of inferior nasal meatus
3. superior nasal concha artery	6. arteries of choanal region	9. inferior nasal concha	12. sphenoidal sinus

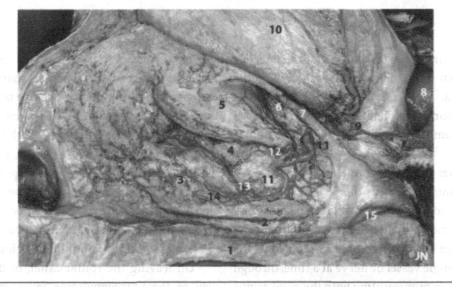

Fig. 79. Right lateral wall of nasal cavity

1. palate	7. superior nasal concha	11. posterior lateral nasal artery	14. inferior nasal concha artery
2. inferior nasal meatus	8. sphenoidal sinus	12. middle nasal concha arteries	15. pharyngeal aperture auditory tube
3. inferior nasal concha	9. septal artery		
4. middle nasal meatus	10. nasal septum (reflected)	13. middle nasal meatus artery	
5. middle nasal concha			
6. superior nasal meatus			

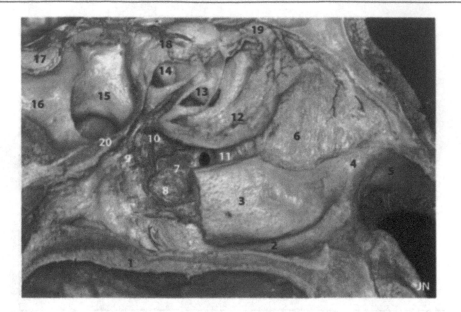

Fig. 80. Left lateral wall of nasal cavity

1. palate	7. middle nasal meatus	11. accessory ostium of maxillary sinus	16. secondary septum of sphenoidal sinus
2. inferior nasal meatus	8. inferior nasal concha artery	12. middle nasal concha	17. hypophysis
3. inferior nasal concha (sectioned)	9. posterior lateral nasal artery	13. ethmoidal bulla	18. posterior ethmoidal artery
4. nasal limen	10. middle nasal concha artery	14. pneumatized superior nasal concha (resected)	19. anterior ethmoidal artery
5. nostril		15. sphenoidal sinus	20. septal artery (resected)
6. aditus of middle nasal meatus			

ing out in its interior, with an anatomical behavior similar to that of the artery supplying the middle nasal concha. Its terminal descending branches reach the floor of the nasal cavity and the nasal crest, anastomosing with the septal terminals (Figs. 75–77).

At the level of the sphenopalatine foramen, the vasculonervous set crosses the wall of the fibrous sac, an extension of the periorbita lining the entire pterygopalatine fossa. In order to avoid leakage of adipose tissue from the fossa, the sac allows the transit of a single vessel or nerve at a time, through small orifices communicating with the nasal cavity.

Figure 74 shows the posterior lateral nasal artery underneath the nasal mucosa, approximately 30 mm distal to the tail of the uncinate process. Note that this artery emerges in the nasal cavity, in the interior of the middle nasal concha, near its end (tail) (Figs. 75–77).

Some palatine vasculonervous pedicles may reach the nasal cavity through the many dehiscences in the vertical plate of the palatine bone, completing its blood supply and innervation. Vasculonervous ends also reach the floor of the nasal cavity through the soft and hard palates, anastomosing with the nasal ends. The same happens with the ends at the tonsillar level, in the nasobuccal transition, where branches of the facial nerve and of the pharyngeal plexus meet, helping to supply these two topographically continuous regions.

On leaving the round canal, in the posterior wall of the pterygopalatine fossa, the maxillary nerve emits communicating branches to the pterygopalatine ganglion in order to maintain the parasympathetic connections. Thereafter, the maxillary nerve leaves the fossa laterally via the pterygomaxillary fissure. Within the zygomatic fossa, it emits posterior superior alveolar branches and the descending palatine branch, continuing anteriorly to the inferior orbital fissure, where it enters the infraorbital groove, together with the homonymous artery.

In the pterygopalatine fossa, maxillary arterial and nervous branches start to pursue a common route, spreading out to the paranasal sinuses, the orbit, and the nasal and oral cavities.

The anterior and posterior ethmoidal branches of the ophthalmic artery, accompanied with the respective nerves, leave the orbit via its medial wall, through the homonymous foramina located at the junction of the frontal and ethmoid bones, which constitute the superior border of this wall. Accessory foramina, if present, are generally found near the posterior foramen, with thin vasculonervous pedicles traversing them. The periorbita protrudes, forming small funnels in order to accommodate the ethmoidal vasculonervous sets in their route through the highly delicate bony canals in a lateromedial and posteroanterior direction. The course of these canals is from the orbit to the surface of the anterior cranial fossa, ending at the level of the lateral and posterolateral edges of the cribriform plate of the ethmoid, respectively (Fig. 81).

The anterior ethmoidal canal is generally single, well-defined and wide, while the posterior is multiple, narrower, and irregularly branched out. Through them and wrapped by the periorbita, the delicate ethmoidal pedicles reach the cranial surface of the cribriform plate. From the orbital side, the anterior and posterior ethmoidal foramina are placed in an anteroposterior sequence. Taking the lacrimal crest as a starting point, they are 24, 12, and 6 mm distant from the optic foramen, respectively.

It is interesting that the origin of the orbital contents and its wrapper, the periorbita, precedes that of the surrounding bony elements. Hence, the ethmoidal cells are situated according to the canals, which vary little in location, course, and dimension. Consequently, the ethmoidal canals are not always related to the roof of the cells but lie at different levels, depending on the degree of cellular expansion. The cranial aperture of the anterior ethmoidal canal is strongly related to the ethmoidal fovea, which protrudes vertically and medially over the cribriform plate of the ethmoid, while the posterior ethmoidal canal and its orbital and cranial foramina may be strongly related to the optic canal, near the orbital vertex, posing severe anatomosurgical risks.

Over the cribriform plate, the thin branches of the ethmoidal arteries and nerves pursue a posteroanterior course, traversing individual cribriform foramina situated among the olfactory foramina in order to reach the nasal roof, septum, and lateral

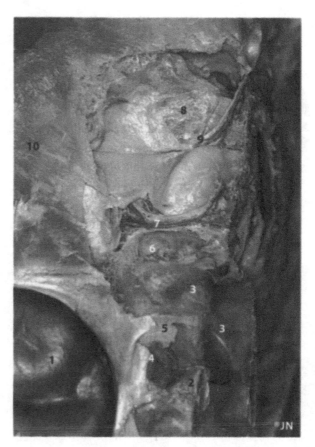

Fig. 81. Cranial view of ethmoidal cells and arteries, left side

1. middle cranial fossa	7. posterior ethmoidal artery
2. hypophysis	
3. sphenoidal sinus	8. anterior ethmoidal cell
4. ophthalmic artery	9. anterior ethmoidal artery
5. optic nerve	
6. posterior ethmoidal cell	10. anterior cranial fossa

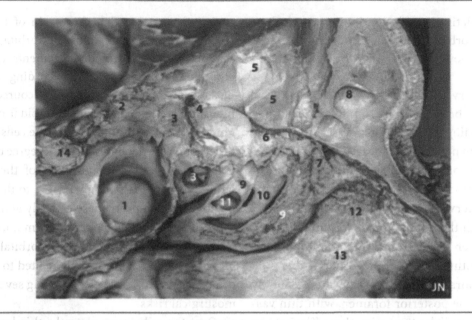

Fig. 82. Cranionasal view of ethmoidal cells and nasal cavity, left side

1. sphenoidal sinus with resected septum	5. anterior ethmoidal cell	9. middle nasal concha (resected)	12. aditus of middle nasal meatus
2. optic nerve	6. anterior ethmoidal artery	10. ethmoidal bulla	13. inferior nasal concha
3. posterior ethmoidal cell	7. middle nasal concha arteries	11. lateral sinus	14. hypophysis
4. posterior ethmoidal artery	8. frontal sinus		

walls. Arterial and nerve branches run anteriorly along the roof and lateral nasal walls to reach internally the nasal dorsum. These are the external ethmoidal branches, which anastomose with the ends of the maxillary and facial arteries and nerves. As previously described, the ethmoidal branches communicate in general with the ones of the nasal cavity, at the most superior level of the septum and nasal walls (Figs. 78–82).

At the most superior part of the septum, the ends of the olfactory nerves and of the ethmoidal arteries become indistinguishable, since they are lodged in a very restricted space, lined by a thick mucous membrane and under the very thin cribriform plate and surrounded by ethmoidal cells, which are often sizable and fragile. The terminal branches of the ethmoidal arteries and nerves reach this region by traversing the cranial surface of the cribriform plate through individual foramina; then they are distributed to the septal pituitary mucosa and the most superior parts of the lateral

wall of the nasal cavity. These thin branches are always subperiosteal and subperichondrial and are difficult to dissect even under magnifying lenses. They are best visualized when injected with silicone or other contrast medium.

The nasopalatine vasculonervous pedicle (Scarpa's pedicle), derived from the septal artery and nerve, descends through the nasal septum bilaterally, close to the superior edge of the vomer, until it reaches the incisive foramina via the nasal floor in the premaxilla. Along this course, the canals merge together, as dothe pedicles therein, exiting in the incisive foramen, in the anterior palate.

Other vasculonervous ends help to supply the septum. The most superior ends anastomose with the homologous ethmoidal ones; the anterior ends communicate with the ones originating from the facial and infraorbital branches, while the descending terminals reach the nasal floor and anastomose with the ones from the palate, constituting the transpalatine communications. Since the nasal

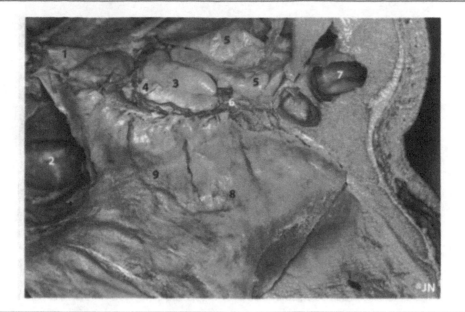

Fig. 83. Cranioseptal view of the ethmoidal cells and arteries, left and right sides

1. optic nerve	4. posterior ethmoidal artery	6. anterior ethmoidal artery	9. septal branches
2. sphenoidal sinus	5. anterior ethmoidal cell	7. frontal sinus	of the posterior
3. posterior ethmoidal cell		8. nasal septum	ethmoidal artery

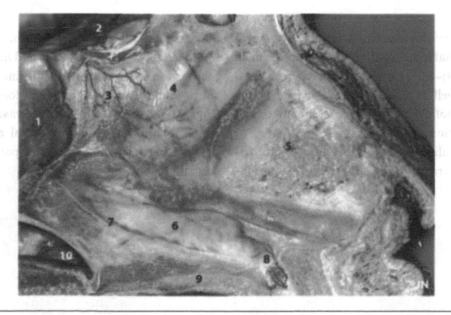

Fig. 84. Arteries of the nasal septum, right side

1. sphenoidal sinus	3. septal branches of the	5. septal cartilage	8. incisive canal
2. anterior cranial fossa	posterior ethmoidal artery	6. vomer	9. palate
	4. ethmoidal perpendicular	7. nasopalatine artery	10. choanal region
	plate	and nerve	

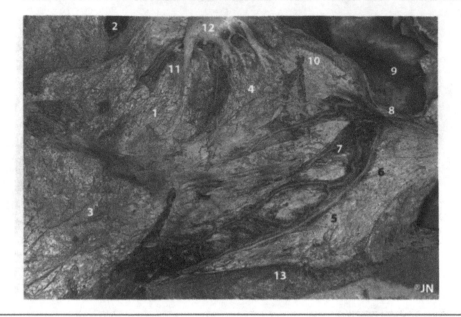

Fig. 85. Nasal septum, left side

1. Nasal septum covered by mucosa	5. vomer	8. site where septal artery reaches nasal septum	11. septal branches of the anterior ethmoidal artery
2. frontal sinus	6. nasopalatine nerve	9. sphenoidal sinus	12. septal ends of olfactory nerve
3. septal cartilage	7. nasopalatine artery and branches	10. septal branches of the posterior ethmoidal artery	13. palate
4. ethmoidal perpendicular plate			

septum is very thin, several arterial anastomoses and transseptal nerve communications occur at all levels (Figs. 83–85). The nerves supplying the nasal septum, as well as those of the other parts of the nasal cavity, follow closely the corresponding arterial ramification.

The vascular plexus of the nasal septum is most concentrated in the superior and anteroin-ferior portions of the septum. Transseptal branches allow a wide vascular and nervous communication that compensates, in most cases, for surgical and traumatic unilateral losses of tissue (Figs. 83–85). Despite the prolific vasculonervous supply of the nasal cavity, several arteries and nerves of facial, infraorbital, and palatine origin contribute to complete it.

Chapter 7
Maxillary Sinus

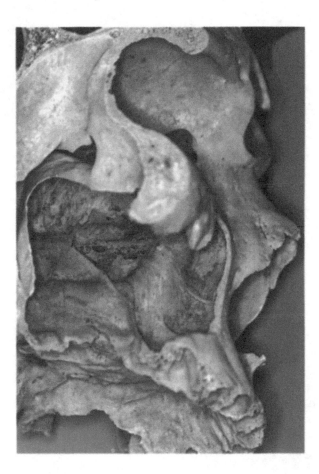

Chapter 7
Maxillary Sinus

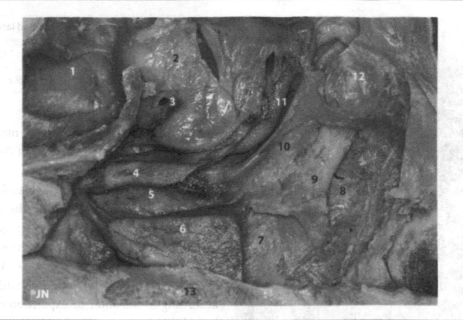

Fig. 86. Left lateral wall of nasal cavity

1. sphenoidal sinus	4. middle nasal concha (resected)	7. inferior nasal meatus	9. nasolacrimal duct
2. posterior ethmoidal cell	5. middle nasal meatus	8. anterior expansion of maxillary sinus (lacrimal)	10. uncinate process
3. ostium of posterior ethmoidal cell	6. inferior nasal concha (resected)		11. ethmoidal bulla
			12. agger nasi
			13. palate

The medial wall of the maxillary sinus projects over the lateral wall of the nasal cavity; its superior border is at the level of the orbital floor, where the infraorbital groove-canal is seen, inclined from posterior to anterior and from medial to lateral, opening at approximately 1 cm from the infraorbital edge. The most concave portion of the posterior wall of the maxillary sinus is near and lateral to the maxillopalatine junction, which corresponds to the anteromedial border of the pterygopalatine fossa. The projection of the sinus floor may be above, at the level of or below the floor of the nasal cavity, depending on such factors as race, sex, age, or function. In the growth phase, there is a dynamic spatial relationship between the orbit, the nasal cavity, the maxillary sinus, and the teeth and their eruptive sequence, varying from the fetus to the adult. The anterior projection of the maxillary sinus over the lateral wall of the nasal cavity varies according to the lacrimal expansion of the maxillary sinus and may be lateral, anterior, or posterior

to the nasolacrimal duct. This is an important anatomical aspect to be considered in the course of a dacryocystorhinostomy using the endonasal approach (Fig. 99).

This large area of sinusal projection extends to the middle nasal meatus and to a large part of the inferior nasal meatus. While the nasal wall of the inferior nasal meatus is thick and harbors solely the ostium of the nasolacrimal duct, the wall of the middle nasal meatus is thin and rich in ethmoidal anatomical elements, also present in the lateral wall of the nasal cavity. The anatomical relationship of the roof of the maxillary sinus with the wall of the middle nasal meatus is variable. The structures of major anatomosurgical importance found in this wall are the uncinate process, the ethmoidal bulla, and the ostia of the ethmoidal and sinusal cells (see Fig. 86).

The main ostium of the maxillary sinus is very close to the sinus roof, as seen from the side of the sinus. It continues as a small canal with an infero-

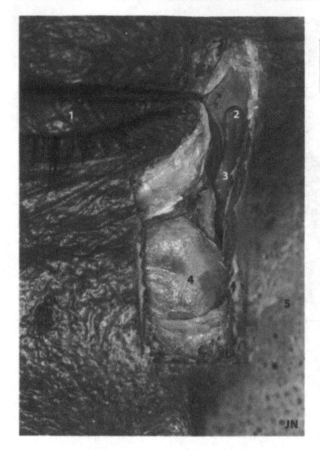

superior and posteroanterior course, to open in the semilunar hiatus, either at the midpoint of the anteroposterior extension of the uncinate process, or in its anterior or posterior one third, according to van Alyea (Figs. 91, 101).

Surgical removal of the uncinate process allows the maxillary sinus to communicate with the ethmoidal cells. Hence, the safest procedure in anterior ethmoidectomies would be access through the ethmoidal bulla. Distal to the uncinate process and the ethmoidal bulla is the wall of the middle nasal meatus, a thin structure, frequently devoid of bony support, occasionally harboring one or more accessory ostia of the maxillary sinus. The posterior space in the transition from the middle to the superior nasal meatus and between the orbital floor and the maxillary sinus may be invaded by posterior or anterior ethmoidal cells, as described by Haller. They are well visible in coronal tomographs (cf. Fig. 122). This region may also accommodate anteroposterior expansions of the sphenoidal si-

nus, competing for space with the maxillary sinus and interfering with the anatomy of the pterygopalatine fossa (Fig. 96).

The uncinate process and the nasolacrimal duct may frequently protrude within the maxillary sinus, the former as a pillar projecting anterior or posterior to the main ostium of the sinus and the latter as a convexity in the medial wall of the sinus, near its anterosuperior junction, which can vary according to the anterior expansion of the maxillary sinus.

The close relationship of the maxillary sinus with the nasolacrimal duct has long been described by Sieur and Jacob, Zuckerkandl, Killian, and more recently Skillern. This anatomical relationship should be considered during surgery involving an endonasal approach, as the lacrimal expansion of the maxillary sinus intervenes between the frontal process of the maxilla and the nasolacrimal duct in varying extension.

The removal of the nasal or the medial wall of the maxillary sinus makes all other walls visible, as well as their anatomical elements. In the specimen shown in Fig. 88, the medial wall of the pterygopalatine fossa was also removed and its vasculonervous contents exposed. In the posterior wall of the maxillary sinus, some posterior superior alveolar vasculonervous branches are observed descending via the endosteum towards the sinus floor, where they will integrate with the superior dental plexus. The curved and concave lateral wall is the largest sinusal projection, termed the zygomatic or pyramidal expansion. Middle superior alveolar vasculonervous branches also run along the lateral wall, reaching the superior dental plexus. The infraorbital canal with its vasculonervous contents is located on the sinus roof; it is often prominent and diverges occasionally from the roof, pursuing a posteroanterior, superoinferior, and mediolateral diagonal course to open in the infraorbital foramen, in the anterior wall of the sinus. Immediately before it opens, the anterior superior alveolar pedicle leaves the canal laterally, surrounds it inferiorly, and takes a medial direction to reach the lateral edge of the piriform aperture, where it turns 90° downward to gain the anterior teeth and periodontium. These are the vasculonervous components of the premaxilla in the fetus. In their diagonal and lateromedial route on the anterior wall of the maxillary sinus, these elements could be damaged in the course of transmaxillary surgical procedures (Fig. 85).

Among the expansions and recesses of the maxillary sinus, the ones of the roof, of the anterior wall, and of the floor pose the highest surgical risks. The risk related to the sinus floor is due to the presence of dental roots of the upper premolars and molars projected within the sinus to a variable extent, depending on the degree of sinusal expansion and factors such as genetic back-

ground, race, age, and traumas (Figs. 89–92). During the growth phase, several changes occur in the sinusal relations, before the common space of the middle face is harmoniously occupied by its respective anatomical elements. Also the posterior (tuberous) wall of the maxillary sinus may present dehiscences due to its variable thickness, with risks for the anatomical relationship with the maxillary artery and its tuberous branches, especially the infraorbital artery, which is very close to the tuberosity, and the periosteal nerve branches (Figs. 93–95).

The nasal wall of the maxillary sinus has a regular anatomy in its inferior two thirds; however, there are recesses and a variable number of ostia near the sinus roof, one of them being the main ostium and the others accessory. The ostia are always located in the free area of the medial nasal meatus and communicate directly with the nasal cavity, presenting diameters varying from 1 to 25 mm (Figs. 87, 88, 92). The main ostium communicates with the nasal cavity via a narrow canal only a few

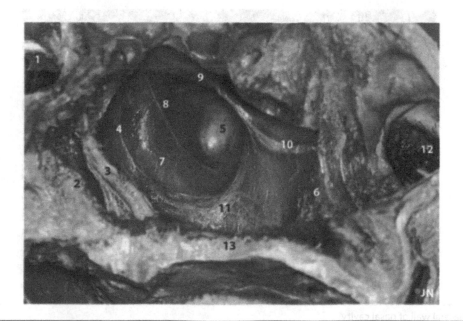

Fig. 88. Left maxillary sinus, dissected by the nasal cavity

1. sphenoidal sinus	4. posterior ⎫	8. middle superior	11. superior dental
2. choanal region	5. lateral ⎬ maxillary sinus walls	alveolar nerve	nervous plexus
3. pterygopalatine fossa, with its vasculonervous elements	6. anterior ⎭ 7. posterior superior alveolar nerve	9. infraorbital canal 10. anterior superior alveolar nerve	12. nostril 13. palate

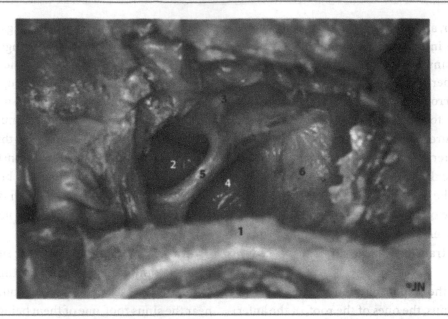

Fig. 89. Right maxillary sinus, opened through the nasal cavity

1. palate	3. maxillary sinus roof	5. diagonal infraorbital canal into the maxillary sinus	6. posterior wall of the maxillary sinus
2. lateral recess (zygomatic) of the maxillary sinus	4. maxillary sinus lateral wall		

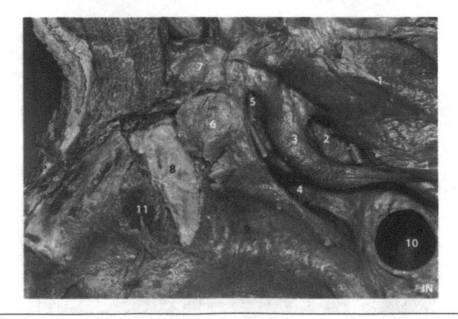

Fig. 90. Right lateral wall of nasal cavity

1. middle nasal concha (reflected)	5. probe in the nasofrontal duct	8. nasolacrimal duct	11. aditus of middle nasal meatus
2. lateral sinus	6. uncinate process (pneumatized)	9. middle nasal meatus	
3. ethmoidal bulla	7. agger nasi cell	10. accessory ostium of maxillary sinus (approximate diameter 15 mm)	
4. semilunar hiatus			

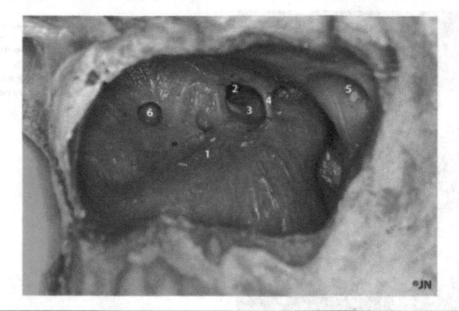

Fig. 91. Lateral view of right maxillary sinus

1. medial wall (nasal)	2. main ostium of maxillary sinus	3. medial recess	5. anterior recess
		4. anterior septum	6. accessory ostium

Fig. 92. Left bony maxillary sinus, anterolateral aperture

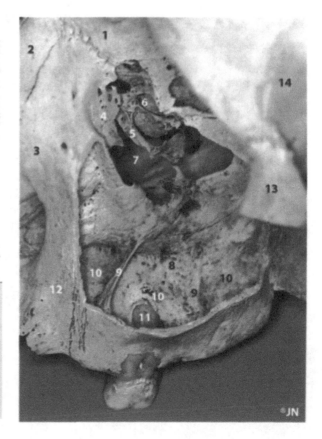

1. frontal	9. bony septa of maxillary sinus
2. nasal	10. sinusal recess
3. frontal process	11. dental root in the floor of the maxillary sinus
4. lacrimal	12. maxilla
5. uncinate process	13. zygomatic frontal process
6. ethmoidal cells	
7. nasal cavity	14. temporal fossa
8. maxillary sinus	

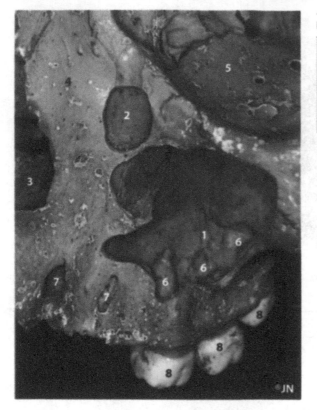

Fig. 93. Bony maxillary sinus, anterolateral aperture, left side

1. maxillary sinus	6. dental roots in the floor
2. anterosuperior recess	of the maxillary sinus
of maxillary sinus	7. dental alveoli
3. nasal cavity	8. maxillary permanent
4. frontal process	molars
5. orbit	

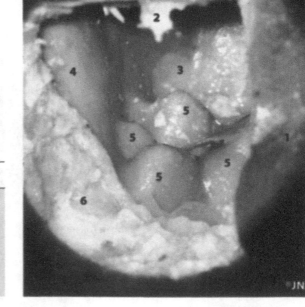

Fig. 94. Maxillary sinus, anterior aperture, right side

1. nose	5. dental roots in the floor
2. infraorbital nerves	of the maxillary sinus
and vessels	6. anterior wall
3. posterior wall	of maxillary sinus
of maxillary sinus	(resected)
4. lateral wall	
of maxillary sinus	

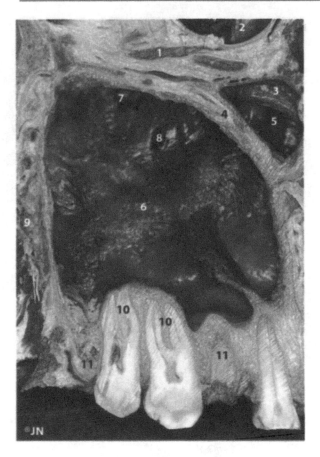

Fig. 95. Lateral view of maxillary sinus, sagittal section, right side

1. orbital floor	8. accessory ostium
2. orbit	of maxillary sinus
3. infraorbital canal	9. pterygopalatine fossa
4. sinusal septum	region
5. sinusal recess	10. dental roots
6. medial (nasal) wall	in the maxillary
of maxillary sinus	sinus floor
7. main ostium	11. alveolar process
of maxillary sinus	of maxillary sinus

millimeters long, with a posteroanterior and inferosuperior course, opening at the deepest portion of the infundibulum canal as the main ostium of the maxillary sinus. Its sinusal aperture is frequently surrounded by fibromucous arches opening inferiorly, as if protecting it or directing its drainage. This wall also has fibrous and bony septa, from which recesses of varying extensions and depths originate. The septa can be so large as to create internal sinusal divisions, wrongly regarded

as the orbitomaxillary cells (Haller). Such recesses, depending on their location, may hamper intranasal surgical procedures (Figs. 88, 89, 91, 100).

Sieur and Jacob, Hajek, Killian, and Terracol and Ardouin refer to a maxillofrontal sinus, as if a single ethmoidal cell gave origin to both sinuses by extending from the maxilla to the frontal bone. In this case, the drainage would be processed from the frontal sinus to the maxillary sinus, and from there to the nasal cavity (cf. Fig. 118).

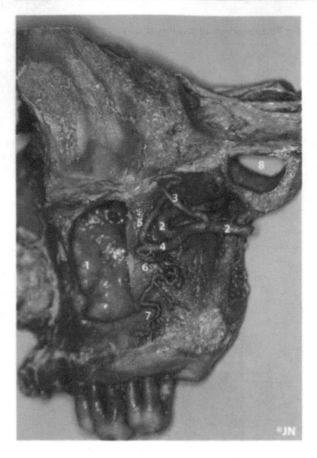

Fig. 96. Maxillary sinus and artery, left side

1. maxillary sinus	5. infraorbital artery
2. maxillary artery	6. posterior superior
3. muscular branch	alveolar artery
of maxillary artery	7. gingival artery
4. posterior superior	8. sphenoidal sinus
infraorbital/alveolar	
branch	

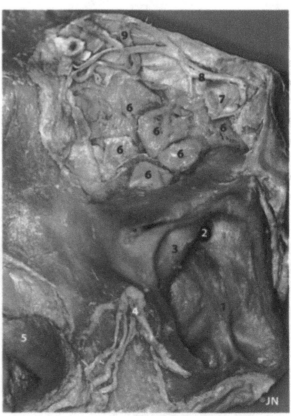

Fig. 97. Maxillary sinus, orbit, and infraorbital canal, left side

1. maxillary sinus	5. nose
2. accessory ostium	6. ethmoidal cells
of maxillary sinus	7. optic nerve (resected)
3. infraorbital canal	8. ophthalmic artery
4. infraorbital artery	9. anterior ethmoidal
and nerve	artery and nerve

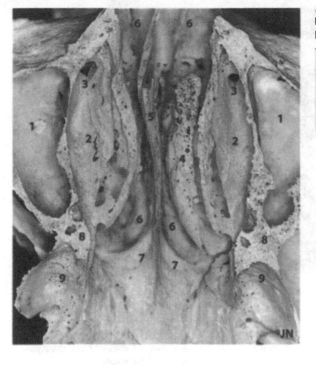

Fig. 98. Inferior view of axial section of the nasal cavity and bony maxillary sinuses, at the level of the inferior nasal concha

1. maxillary sinus	5. nasal septum
2. inferior nasal meatus	6. superior nasal wall
3. nasal opening of the nasolacrimal duct	7. ala of vomer
	8. pterygoid process
4. middle nasal concha	9. pterygoid fossa

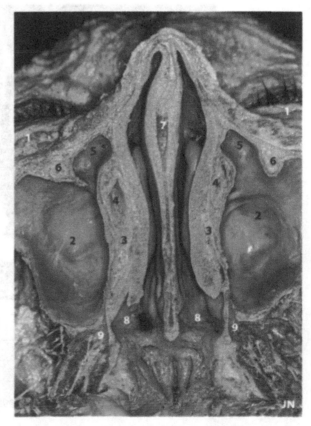

Fig. 99. Inferior view of axial section of the nasal cavity and maxillary sinuses, at the level of the inferior nasal concha

1. eyelid region	6. infraorbital canal
2. maxillary sinus	7. nasal septum
3. inferior nasal concha	8. choanal region
4. nasolacrimal duct	9. pterygopalatine region
5. maxillary sinus lacrimal recess	

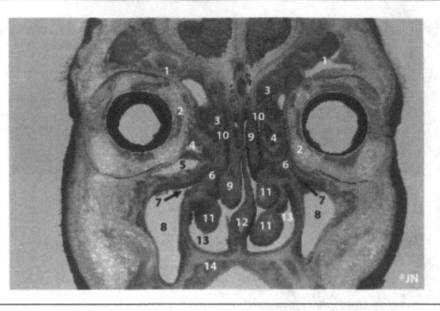

Fig. 100. Coronal section at mid level of the nasal cavity

1. frontal sinus	5. orbitomaxillary cell (Haller)	8. maxillary sinus	12. nasal septum
2. orbit	6. uncinate process	9. middle nasal concha	13. inferior nasal meatus
3. ethmoidal cells	7. maxillary duct and ostium (arrows)	10. middle nasal meatus	14. palate
4. ethmoidal bulla		11. inferior nasal concha	

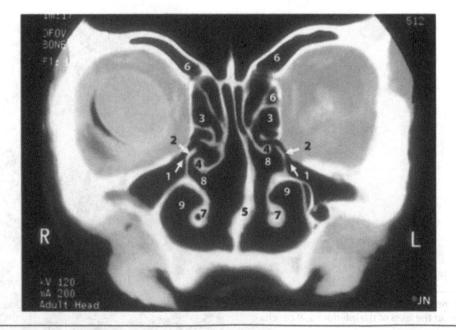

Fig. 101. Coronal CT section at mid level of the nasal cavity

1. duct and ostium of maxillary sinus (arrows)	3. ethmoidal bulla	5. nasal septum	8. middle nasal meatus
2. uncinate process	4. middle nasal concha	6. ethmoidal cells	9. inferior nasal meatus
		7. inferior nasal concha	

(Reproduced with thanks from Dr. Rainer Haetinger, Med Imagem, São Paulo, Brazil)

Chapter 8
Frontal Sinus

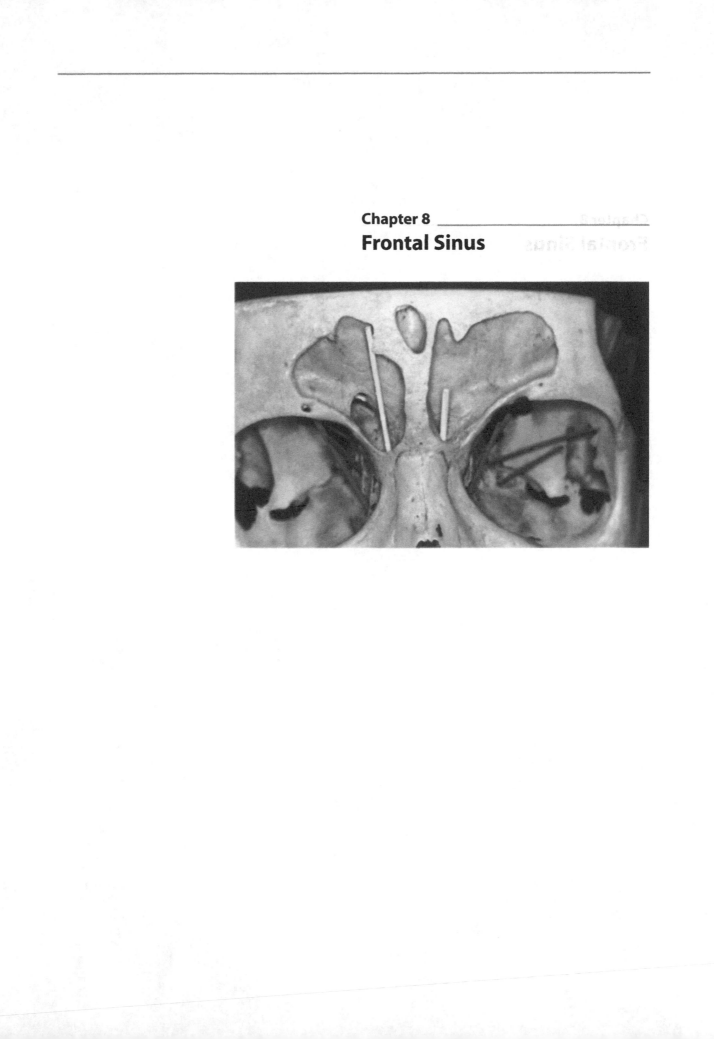

Chapter 8
Frontal Sinus

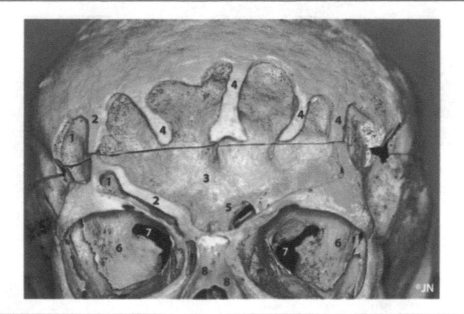

Fig. 102. Wide bony frontal sinus, anterior dissection

1. right frontal sinus
2. main septum
  of frontal sinus
	3. left frontal sinus
	4. accessory septa
	  of the left frontal sinus
		5. frontonasal recess
		  of the left frontal sinus
		6. orbit
			7. superior orbital fissure
			8. nasal

At the end of the fetal stage, the most anterior ethmoidal cells, still very small, are located near the hemifrontal orbital region, separated by the interfrontal or the metopic sutural space. These cells are lodged in soft connective tissue structures as individual epithelial invaginations. If a sinusal agenesis does not occur, after the second postnatal year at least one of these cells at either side will reach the frontal bone. By the fourth year, they are already radiographically detectable. From an embryological point of view, this sinus displays important and peculiar features with respect to the site in the nasal cavity where it opens and drains. The site of origin of every paranasal sinus in the nasal epithelium will also be the place where its drainage ostia will be. Wherever a cavity begins, it will grow in a genetically programmed fashion to occupy the most diverse anatomical areas, within the ethmoid itself or in the bones harboring other sinuses (Fig. 102). For the frontal sinus, the original cells may be, from the beginning, very close to the base of the frontal bone or expand in other directions. In the first case, an ethmoidal cell enters the frontal bone directly via a wide frontonasal ostium, without the need of a duct, starting its pneumatization. However, if the cell is formed at a distance, in its route of expansion to the frontal bone it has to pass through other cells, being compressed and deformed by the time it arrives. This is how the duct is formed, i.e., as an extension of the original ostium in the nasal wall.

The systematization of this anatomical behavior remains a challenge. Further studies focusing craniofacial morphofunctional and dysfunctional aspects may contribute to a better understanding of the nasosinus complex.

Among the cells initiating the frontal pneumatization, two are basic and give origin to the left and right sinuses. Other cells may expand, but they are usually of small volume and remain minor to the main ones, or lateralize to larger proportions. These are the cells described by Boyer and Zuckerkandl in the nineteenth century (Figs. 103, 104). It is important that each cell has its own ostium, otherwise it will be considered an extension of another cell.

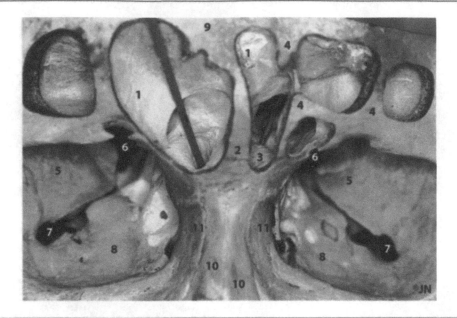

Fig. 103. Bony frontal sinuses, anterior dissection

1. frontal sinuses (probes into the sinusal recesses)	3. ethmoidal cell (frontal bulla)	5. orbit	9. frontal
2. main septum of frontal sinus, with left deviation	4. accessory septa of frontal sinus	6. superior orbital fissure	10. nasal
		7. inferior orbital fissure	11. maxillary frontal process
		8. orbital floor	

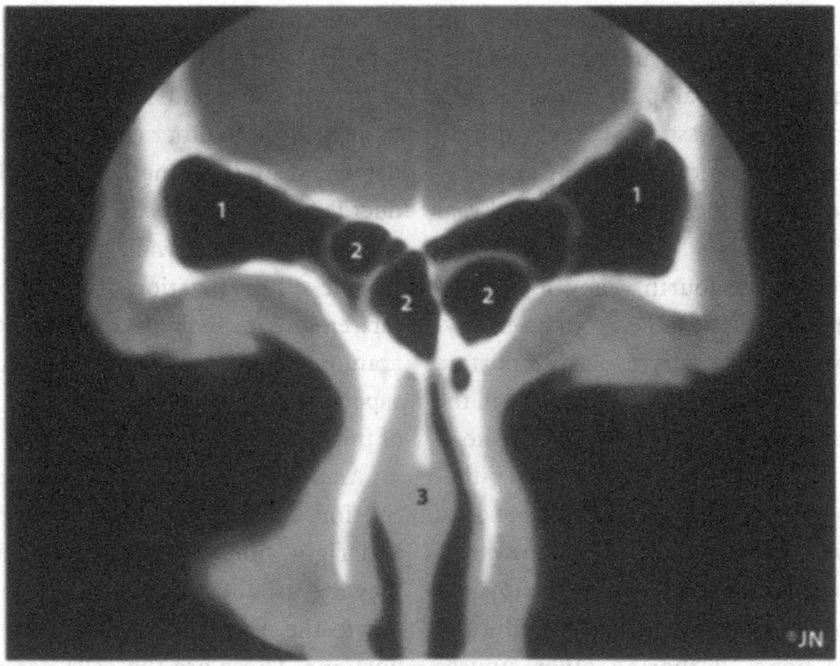

Fig. 104. Coronal CT of the nasal cavity and frontal sinuses with bilateral frontal bulla

1. frontal sinus	2. frontal bullae	3. nasal septum

(Reproduced with thanks from Dr. Rainer Haetinger, Med Imagem, São Paulo, Brazil)

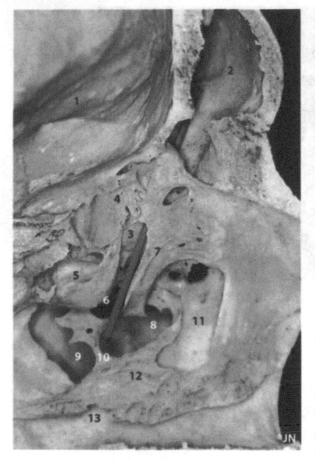

Fig. 105. Bony frontonasal duct, left side

1. anterior cranial fossa	8. anterior window
2. frontal sinus	9. posterior window
3. frontonasal duct (probe)	10. ethmoidal process
4. agger nasi	of inferior nasal concha
5. ethmoidal bulla	11. nasolacrimal duct
6. semilunar hiatus	12. inferior nasal concha
7. uncinate process	13. inferior nasal meatus

(16%). The existence, extension, and diameter of the drainage duct depends on the (genetically determined) site of origin of the cell. This is an area of great surgical risk, owing to the proximity of the ostium or the duct of the frontal sinus to the anterior cranial fossa and particularly to the cribriform plate of the ethmoid and ethmoidal fovea. The complex anatomical relationship of this area with the perilacrimal ethmoidal cells adds to this risk.

The frontal sinuses have as bony borders the crista galli process, the intersinusal septum from the cranial side, and the nasal septum from the side of the nasal cavity. Their base, like the base of the anterior ethmoidal cells, is in the interorbital and supraorbital spaces.

The agger nasi cells are located medial to the drainage site of the frontal sinus, somewhat below it and in close relation to the lacrimal sac and the most superior part of the nasolacrimal duct. Some frontal cells may pneumatize the crista galli, thereby occupying more anterior spaces.

The anterosuperior region of the nasal cavity, where the ethmoidal and frontal ostia are found, is extremely narrow due to the presence of the nasal septum and the convergence of the frontal processes of the maxilla and their nasofrontal junction (Fig. 105). The extreme anterior placement of these structures in relation to the nasal aditus render the endonasal access to the most anterior cells and to the frontal sinus quite difficult. Hence, it is important for the surgeon to have a precise knowledge of the drainage sites of the sinus and cells and their anatomical relationship with the base of the cranium, in order to avoid bone traumas resulting in fistulae (Figs. 103–105).

At the meeting point of the two basic cells within the frontal bone, a main bony septum will remain, separating them completely. The position of this septum varies according to the (genetically determined) cellular anatomy, the bony resistance to pneumatization, and the air pressure. This septum is seldom in the median plane and hardly ever vertical, except in its most inferior one third or one fourth, near the base of the sinus. Accessory, partial or incomplete septa may be observed starting at the sinus walls, varying greatly in number, position, and dimension (Figs. 102–104).

An orbitonasal base and two walls – an anterior and a posterior – give this sinus its triangular aspect, with lateral projections in parietal, posterior, supraorbital, ethmoid, and sphenoid directions.

The drainage ostium of the cell pneumatizing the frontal bone remains at the cell's site of origin; this can be the frontoethmoidal recess (47%), the infundibulum (37%), or the prebullar region

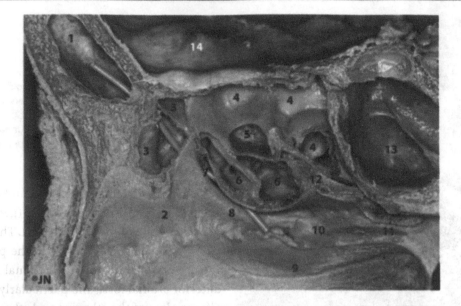

Fig. 106. Right lateral wall of nasal cavity

1. Probe into the frontal sinus, anterior ethmoidal cell, and infundibulum, emerging by the uncinate process	2. aditus of middle nasal meatus 3. anterior ethmoidal cells 4. posterior ethmoidal cells 5. suprabullar anterior cell 6. ethmoidal bulla	7. semilunar hiatus, reduced by the ethmoidal bulla 8. uncinate process 9. inferior nasal concha 10. middle nasal meatus 11. choanal region	12. middle nasal concha (resected) 13. sphenoidal sinus 14. anterior cranial fossa

The supraorbital expansions of the frontal sinus may resemble an anterior ethmoidal cell. In fact, the ethmoidal cell forming the frontal sinus can emerge from different areas of the nasoethmoidal complex, extending to supraorbital and interorbital spaces and even to the parietal regions. According to Zuckerkandl, the frontal sinus may occasionally take its origin in the sphenoethmoidal recess. The right and left nasal apertures of the frontal sinus are always separated by the nasal septum. A variable number of ethmoidal cells may reach the frontal sinus, but only two of them will initiate the sinuses. The others will compete for space, remaining at the base of the sinus or extending elsewhere (Figs. 106–112).

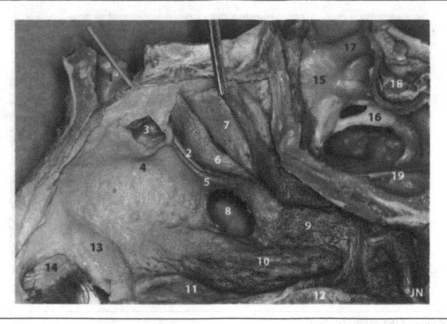

Fig. 107. Right lateral wall of nasal cavity

1. Probe penetrates the frontal sinus and emerges in the semilunar hiatus	5. uncinate process	9. middle nasal meatus	14. nostril
2. semilunar hiatus	6. ethmoidal bulla	10. inferior nasal concha	15. sphenoidal sinus
3. agger nasi cell	7. middle nasal concha (reflected)	11. inferior nasal meatus	16. round canal
4. aditus of middle nasal meatus	8. accessory ostium of maxillary sinus	12. palate	17. optic nerve
		13. nasal limen	18. hypophyseal fossa
			19. pterygoid canal

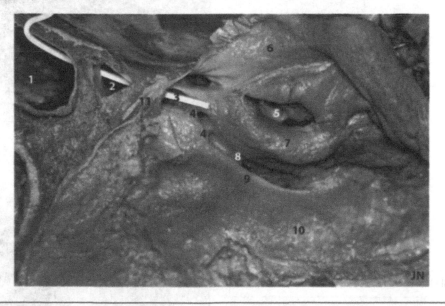

Fig. 108. Right lateral wall of nasal, with exposition of the frontonasal recess and middle nasal meatus

1. Probe traverses the frontal sinus (1) and ethmoidal anterior cell and emerges in the infundibulum	3. infundibulum	6. middle nasal concha (reflected)	10. middle nasal meatus
2. ethmoidal anterior cell	4. ostia cells of middle nasal meatus	7. ethmoidal bulla	11. external nasal artery and nerve
	5. lateral sinus	8. semilunar hiatus	
		9. uncinate process	

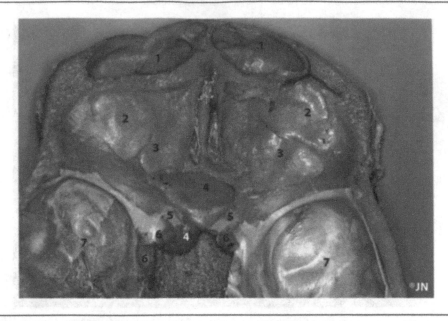

Fig. 109. Cranial view of the paranasal sinus

1. frontal sinus	3. posterior ethmoidal cell	5. optic nerve	7. middle cranial fossa
2. anterior ethmoidal cell	4. sphenoidal sinus	6. internal carotid artery	

Fig. 110. Cranial view of the orbit and paranasal sinuses

1. frontal sinus	7. anterior cranial fossa
2. anterior ethmoidal cell	8. sphenoidal sinus
3. orbit	9. optic nerve
4. posterior ethmoidal cell	10. middle cranial fossa
5. anterior ethmoidal canal	
6. posterior ethmoidal canal	

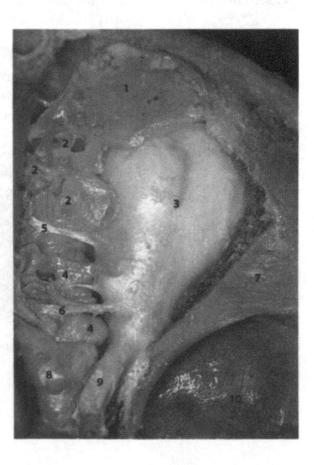

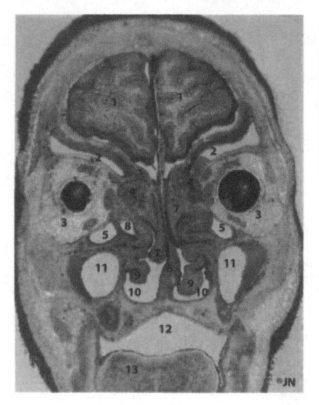

Fig. 111. Coronal section at the mid level of the nasal cavity

1. brain	7. middle nasal concha
2. frontal sinus, supraorbital expansion	8. ethmoidal bulla
	9. inferior nasal concha
3. orbit	10. inferior nasal meatus
4. ethmoidal cells	11. maxillary sinus
5. orbitomaxillary ethmoidal cell (Haller)	12. oral cavity
	13. tongue
6. nasal septum, with deviation	

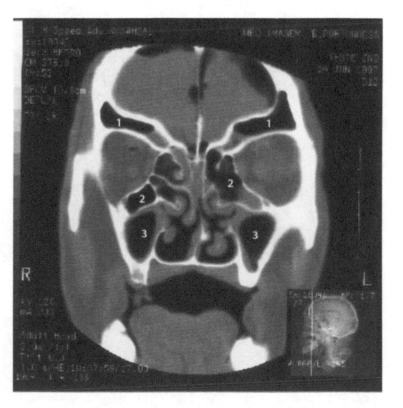

Fig. 112. Coronal CT at the mid level of the nasal cavity

1. frontal sinus with supraorbital expansion
2. orbitomaxillary ethmoidal cell (Haller)
3. maxillary sinus

Chapter 9
Ethmoidal Sinus

Chapter 9 _____
Ethmoidal Sinus

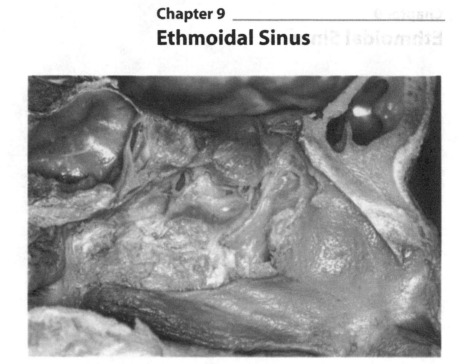

Chapter 9 _____
Ethmoidal Sinus

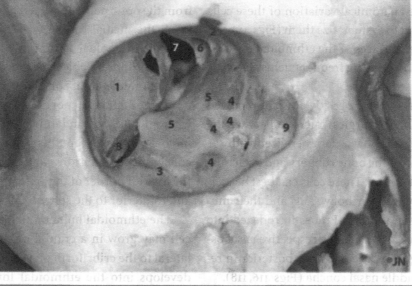

Fig. 113. Orbital view of the ethmoidal cells, right side

1. lateral orbital wall	4. anterior ethmoidal cells	6. optic foramen	8. inferior orbital fissure
2. orbital roof	5. posterior ethmoidal cells	7. superior orbital fissure	9. lacrimal fossa
3. orbital floor			

The orbit is surrounded almost entirely by bones pneumatized by the paranasal sinuses. Over the orbit are the frontal ethmoidal sinuses; under it is the maxillary sinus, and medial is the ethmoidal sinus. The sphenoidal sinus and the orbital process of the palatine bone, generally pneumatized by one or more posterior ethmoidal cells, are at the level of the orbital vertex. The vasculonervous structures penetrating and surrounding the orbit are subject to the same anatomical changes, traumas, and diseases that affect the periorbital regions.

The orbital contents are enveloped by the periorbita, an extension of the dura mater. The same is true of all other intra- and interosseous communications within this cavity. The paranasal sinuses precede in origin the bony structures in which they are contained; hence the bones are shaped by the sinuses, as are the vasculonervous pedicles and the round, optic, infraorbital, and ethmoidal canals.

The medial surface of the orbit (or orbital surface of the ethmoid-papyracea lamina) is in almost total contact with the ethmoidal cells by its walls or orbital borders. The orbital pressure on the perior-

bita keeps its bony surfaces regular, in most cases without prominences or exostoses. In the ethmoido-maxillary junction some cellular expansions may occur, mainly in the most posterior region, where the orbitomaxillary cells (Haller cells) would be (see Figs. 111, 112). The orbital surfaces of the ethmoidal cells are quite thin, making the intercellular septa even more evident. A view through the orbit reveals that the cells closest to the lacrimal region are smaller than those posterior to it (Figs. 113, 116, 117). Actually, a cell may appear small from the orbital side but expand irregularly in other directions, reaching great volume. Some cells do not present an orbital surface, since they are within the ethmoidal complex and related to other surfaces such as the cranial, lacrimal, maxillary, palatine, sphenoidal, frontal, and certainly the nasal cavity.

Classically, the ethmoidal cells are divided into anterior and posterior, according to the placement of their drainage ostium. This division is made by the basal lamella of the middle nasal concha. The anterior ethmoidal cells are considered to be more numerous but smaller in volume, while the posterior cells are lesser in number but more volumi-nous. The wide anatomical variation of these cells makes it difficult to systematize them (Figs. 113, 116, 117). The orbital surfaces of the ethmoidal cells are often very thin, displaying frequent dehiscences, as described in the literature.

These cellular walls are relatively easily removed by dissection under a surgical microscope when the anatomical piece has been demineralized with 5% nitric acid, making the bone rubbery and detaching it from the endosteum. These cells can best be ana-lyzed by removing their bony walls and their mu-cosal and endosteal lining. Probes introduced into the cellular openings reach the respective nasal os-tia, identifying them as anterior or posterior in re-lation to the middle nasal concha (Figs. 116, 118).

In the fetus and during the first two years of life, the ethmoidal cells expand freely; neither is there competition for space between them nor are they yet too close to the cranial or the orbital surfaces. The morphological changes increase with growth, as they become more crowded together and closer to the other sinuses and bony borders.

The ophthalmic arteries and nerves deflect from the optic nerve (resected in this specimen) to reach the medial orbital wall, pursuing a course near the ethmoidal foramina, to which they will send anterior and posterior branches (Fig. 116).

The middle nasal concha is inserted in the su-perior and anterior portions of the nasal cavity, where the cribriform lamina joins the lateral eth-moidal complex. From this point, the middle nasal concha bends inferiorly and posteriorly to reach the inferior border of the sphenopalatine foramen, anteroinferior to the sphenoidal sinus.

The ethmoidal bulla or an anterior ethmoidal cell may grow in a cranial direction and project lateral to the cribriform plate of the ethmoid. This develops into the ethmoidal fovea and changes the vertical distance between the cribriform plate and the supraorbital level, which can reach 16 mm, according to Keros. In extreme cases, the difference in levels may reach up to 21 mm.

The ethmoidal bulla grows cranially between the middle nasal concha and the orbital wall, occa-sionally reaching a level above the cribriform plate.

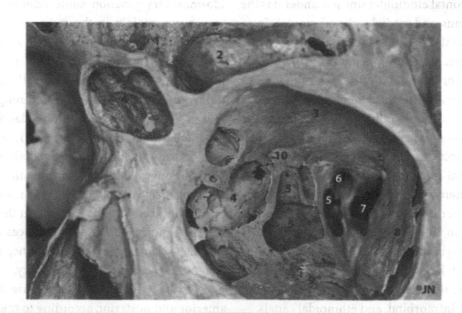

Fig. 114. Ethmoidal cells with their orbital walls removed, left side

1. frontal sinus	3. orbital roof	6. optic foramen	9. orbital floor
2. ethmoidofrontal cell (frontal bulla)	4. anterior ethmoidal cell	7. superior orbital fissure	10. anterior ethmoidal foramen
	5. posterior ethmoidal cell	8. lateral orbital wall	

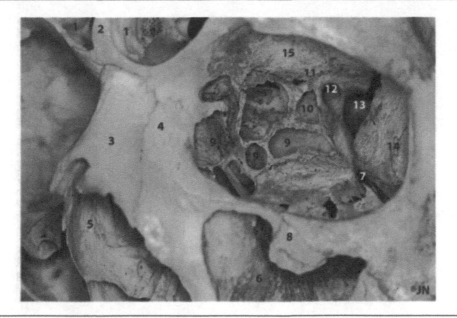

Fig. 115. Ethmoidal cells, with their orbital walls removed, left side

1. frontal sinus	5. nasal cavity	9. anterior ethmoidal cell	12. optic foramen
2. frontal sinus, main septum	6. maxillary sinus	10. posterior ethmoidal cell	13. superior orbital fissure
3. nasal	7. inferior orbital fissure	11. posterior ethmoidal	14. orbital lateral wall
4. maxillary frontal process	8. infraorbital foramen	foramen	15. orbital roof

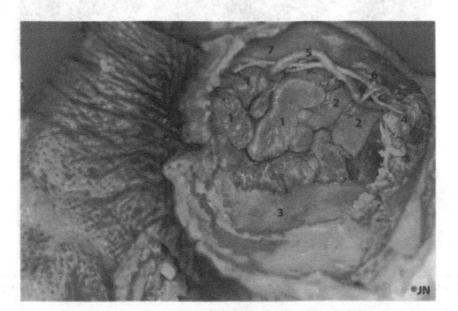

Fig. 116. Ethmoidal cell dissected by the orbit, left side

1. group of anterior ethmoidal cells	2. group of ethmoidal posterior cells	4. sectioned optic nerve	6. nasociliary nerve
	3. orbital floor	5. ophthalmic artery	7. anterior ethmoidal vasculonervous pedicle

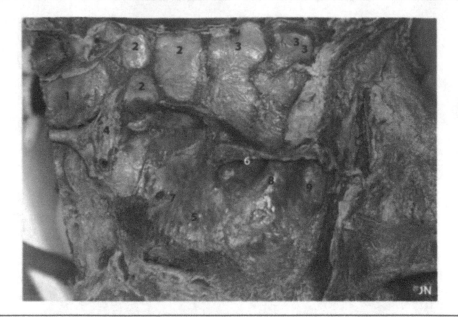

Fig. 117. Sagittal section showing an orbital view of the ethmoidal cells and a lateral view of the maxillary sinus, right side

1. sphenoidal sinus (main septum)	3. group of anterior ethmoidal cells	6. maxillary sinus roof	8. sinusal salience of the nasolacrimal duct
2. group of posterior ethmoidal cells	4. pterygopalatine fossa	7. maxillary sinus, accessory ostium	9. maxillary sinus, anterior (lacrimal) recess
	5. maxillary sinus, nasal (medial) wall		

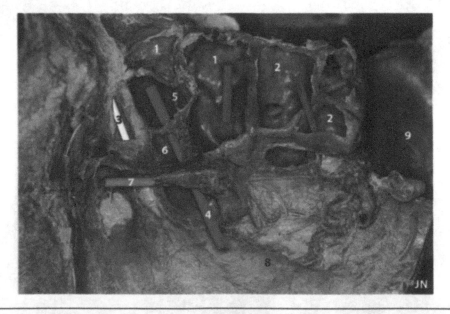

Fig. 118. Sagittal section of the maxillary sinus and ethmoidal cells opened through the orbit and the maxillary sinus, left side

1. group of anterior ethmoidal cells	4. probe (orange) crosses the frontal sinus (5), an anterior ethmoidal cell (6), and emerges in the maxillary sinus	7. probe (green) penetrates main ostium of the maxillary sinus	8. maxillary sinus medial (nasal) wall, sinusal view
2. group of posterior ethmoidal cells			9. sphenoidal sinus
3. probe (white) into the nasolacrimal duct			

The more voluminous the ethmoidal bulla, the thinner and more dehiscent are its walls, according to such authors as Keros and Onishi.

The cranial view in Fig. 120 shows the medial and cranial projections of two anterior ethmoidal cells bilaterally over the cribriform lamina, with probes introduced in the anterior ethmoidal ducts. Foveae and cellular projections to the olfactory areas can also be observed.

In the coronal segment of the head (Fig. 117), at the level of the middle one third of the nasal cavity, the most superior point of insertion of the middle nasal concha is observed, together with the cellular expansions located cranial to the cribriform plate. The interorbitomaxillary cells (Haller cells) can also be seen bilaterally. The duct of the maxillary sinus is found between one of these cells, the ethmoidal bulla and the uncinate process. In this specimen, the uncinate process is compressed by the septum, which is slightly deflected to the right. The left nasal concha is bullous in its most superior portion. The fovea is bilateral and in a much higher position than the cribriform plate of the ethmoid. The left inferior nasal concha is large inside the nasal cavity, which in turn is also wide on the left. The right middle nasal concha is more lateral and its inferior portion is juxtaposed to the uncinate process. On the right side is the duct connecting the sinusal and nasal ostia of the maxillary sinus.

There is still no general agreement in the literature about the location, frequency, and drainage site of the orbitomaxillary cells described by Haller. They originate either in the middle or in the superior nasal meatus; they can be single or multiple but are two on average, and their drainage site depends on their origin. They are nearly always locat-

ed under the orbit and above the maxillary sinus (Figs. 120–122). They seem to be cells originating with the pneumatization of the orbital process of the palatine bone by the most posterior ethmoidal cells. The orbitomaxillary cells can be observed in the skull; however, in the cadaver and in the living the sinusal mucosa renders them imperceptible.

The orbitomaxillary region near the inferior orbital fissure is anatomically complex due to the junction of the ethmoid, sphenoid, maxilla, and palatine bones. Since this region can be thoroughly pneumatized, it is difficult to establish the exact relationship between its various osseous structures. The common posterior area – the pterygopalatine fossa – is frequently compressed by cellular expansions of the neighboring bones. A cellular overgrowth towards the maxillary sinus can reduce the surgical area of the posterior wall of this sinus, hindering the transmaxillary access to the maxillary artery (Fig. 118). The sphenoidal sinus can also expand anteroinferiorly, thus reaching the maxillary sinus and reducing the space for the pterygopalatine fossa.

All paranasal sinuses have their origin in the ethmoidal portion of the nasal cavity. Their com-

Fig. 119. Cranial view of the ethmoidal cells, opened, in relation to the ethmoid cribriform plate

1. frontal sinus	5. probe emerging from
2. anterior ethmoidal cell	the anterior ethmoidal
3. crista galli	foramen, above
4. ethmoidal cribriform	the cribriform plate
plate	6. posterior ethmoidal cell

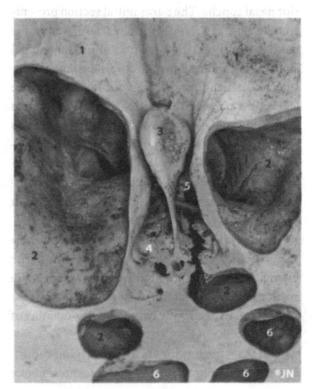

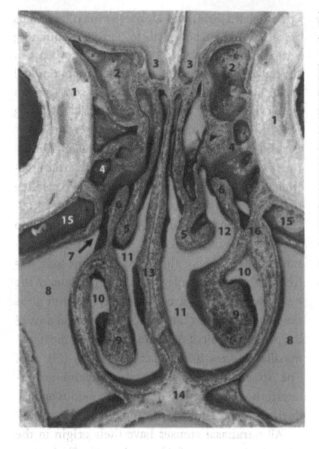

Fig. 120. Coronal view of the ethmoidal cells in relation to the ethmoidal cribriform plate; coronal section at the level of the nasal cavity

1. orbit	8. maxillary sinus
2. anterior ethmoidal cell, with its roof over the ethmoidal cribriform plate's level	9. inferior nasal concha
	10. inferior nasal meatus
	11. common nasal meatus
3. ethmoidal cribriform plate	12. middle nasal meatus
	13. nasal septum
4. ethmoidal bulla	14. palate
5. middle nasal concha	15. ethmoidal orbito-maxillary cells (Haller)
6. uncinate process	16. infundibular canal
7. maxillary sinus, main ostium	

munication with the nasal cavity is above the inferior nasal concha. The parasagittal section presented here (Fig. 123), tangent to the lateral wall of the nasal cavity, shows the open frontal and sphenoidal sinuses. The main septa of both sinuses may be visualized, depending on their position and on the level of the parasagittal section. The nasal surfaces of the ethmoidal cells have been cut away in this section, allowing a direct view of their drainage ostia and of their anatomy and dimensions. The middle and superior nasal conchae were partially resected, but the lamellae and their base of insertion in the nasal wall were left untouched.

The middle meatus is entirely exposed to show the accessory ostium of the maxillary sinus. The uncinate process is totally preserved because the section was not so lateral as to reach it. The agger nasi region was partially exposed by the opening of one of its cells.

Note that the prominence of this region continues in the uncinate process, whose anterior one

third seems to be pneumatized. The ethmoidal bulla is not very voluminous; the nasal wall of its anterior portion was resected (Figs. 124, 125).

The recess or lateral sinus above the bulla is narrow and harbors the ostia of the anterior ethmoidal cells. Probes were introduced into the ostia of the cells and of the maxillary sinus. The probe inside the frontal sinus runs through its ostium or duct and through the frontoethmoidal recess and infundibulum, exiting into the semilunar hiatus. The superior meatus is narrow and elongated; over it lies the tail of the superior nasal concha, extending to the sphenoidal rostrum. A large posterior cell (Onodi cell) is present with a small sphenoethmoidal recess. The sphenoidal sinus is wide and saddle-shaped; a probe crosses its ostium, located at the junction of the middle and the superior thirds (Fig. 125).

Some anatomical variations in the lateral wall of the nasal cavity and the paranasal sinuses are shown in Figs. 120–128; see also Fig. 129.

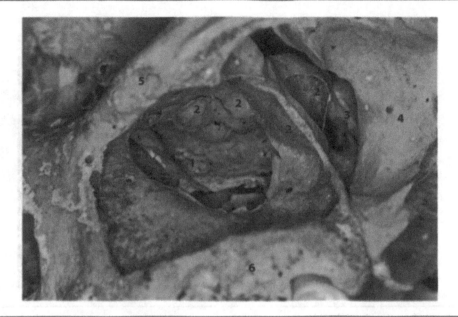

Fig. 121. Left bony maxillary sinus, opened laterally

1. maxillary sinus	2. ethmoidal orbitomaxillary cells (Haller)	3. pterygopalatine fossa 4. pterygoid process	5. zygomatic 6. maxillary alveolar process

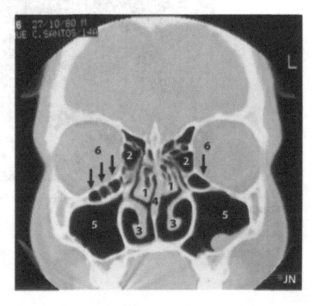

Fig. 122. Coronal CT of the nasal cavity and paranasal sinuses

1. middle bullous nasal concha	4. nasal septum
2. ethmoidal bulla	5. maxillary sinus
3. inferior nasal concha	6. orbitomaxillary (Haller) ethmoidal cells (*arrows*).

(Reproduced with thanks to Dr. R.M. Neves Pinto, Rio de Janeiro, Brazil)

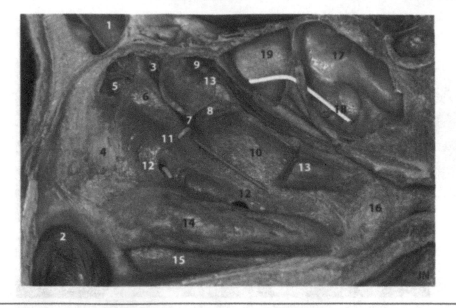

Fig. 123. Lateral wall of nasal cavity, right side

1. frontal sinus	6. uncinate process	12. accessory ostium of maxillary sinus	17. sphenoidal sinus
2. nasal limen	7. semilunar hiatus	13. middle nasal concha (resected)	18. probe (white) in ostium of sphenoidal sinus
3. anterior ethmoidal cells	8. ethmoidal bulla	14. inferior nasal concha	19. posterior ethmoidal cell
4. aditus of middle nasal meatus	9. lateral sinus	15. inferior nasal meatus	
5. agger nasi	10. middle nasal meatus	16. choanal region	
	11. probe (yellow) in main ostium of maxillary sinus		

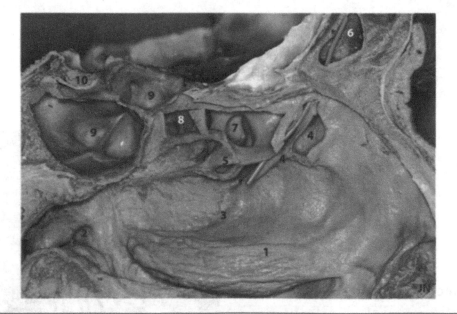

Fig. 124. Lateral wall of nasal cavity, left side

1. inferior nasal concha	3. middle nasal meatus	6. probe introduced into the frontal sinus emerges into the semilunar hiatus	8. posterior ethmoidal cell
2. pharyngeal aperture of auditory tube	4. uncinate process	7. anterior ethmoidal cell	9. sphenoidal sinus
	5. ethmoidal bulla		10. hypophysis

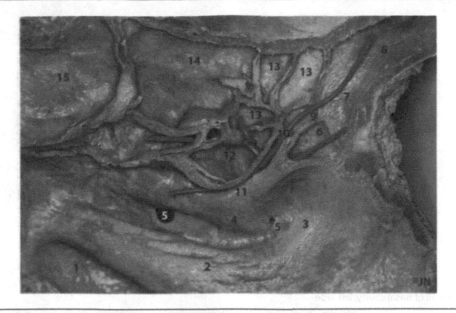

Fig. 125. Lateral wall of nasal cavity, left side

1. inferior nasal meatus	6. pneumatized uncinate	10. infundibulum	14. posterior ethmoidal cell
2. inferior nasal concha	process	11. semilunar hiatus	(Onodi)
3. aditus of middle meatus	7. probe traverses:	12. hypertrophied ethmoidal	15. sphenoidal sinus,
4. middle nasal meatus	8. frontal sinus	bulla obstructs	main septum
5. maxillary sinus,	9. agger nasi cell	the semilunar hiatus	
accessory ostium		13. anterior ethmoidal cell	

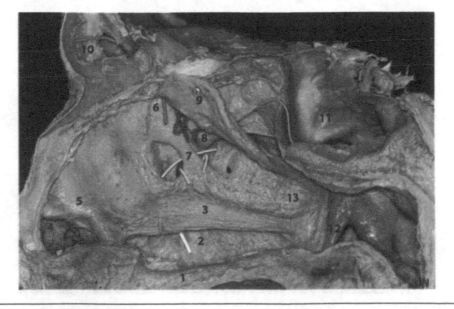

Fig. 126. Nasal cavity's lateral wall, right side

1. palate	5. nasal limen	9. middle nasal concha	12. pharyngeal aperture
2. inferior nasal meatus	6. agger nasi	(reflected)	of auditory tube
3. inferior nasal concha	7. uncinate process	10. frontal sinus	13. middle nasal meatus
4. nostril	8. ethmoidal bulla	11. sphenoidal sinus	

Probes: frontal sinus/agger nasi (orange) anterior ethmoidal cells (red) uncinate process and maxillary sinus ostia (yellow) posterior ethmoidal cell (blue) sphenoid sinus (purple) nasolacrimal duct (white)

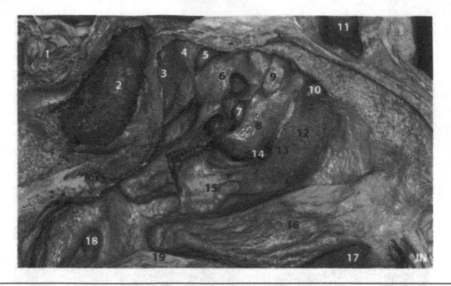

Fig. 127. Lateral wall of nasal cavity, left side

1. hypophysial fossa	6. bullar middle nasal concha (resected)	10. agger nasi cell	15. middle nasal meatus
2. sphenoidal sinus	7. lateral sinus	11. frontal sinus	16. inferior nasal concha
3. sphenoethmoidal recess	8. ethmoidal bulla	12. aditus of middle nasal meatus	17. inferior nasal meatus
4. superior nasal concha	9. prebullous anterior ethmoidal cell	13. uncinate process	18. pharyngeal aperture of auditory tube
5. superior nasal meatus		14. semilunar hiatus	19. palate

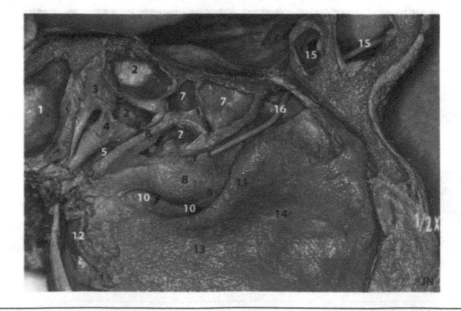

Fig. 128. Lateral wall of nasal cavity, left side

1. sphenoidal sinus	6. lamella of middle nasal concha	10. accessory ostium of maxillary sinus	14. aditus of middle nasal meatus
2. posterior ethmoidal cell	7. anterior ethmoidal cells	11. uncinate process	15. frontal sinus, with a *probe* emerging from an agger nasi cell (16)
3. supreme nasal concha	8. ethmoidal bulla	12. posterior nasolateral artery	
4. superior nasal concha	9. semilunar hiatus	13. middle nasal meatus	
5. superior nasal meatus			

Chapter 10
Sphenoidal Sinus

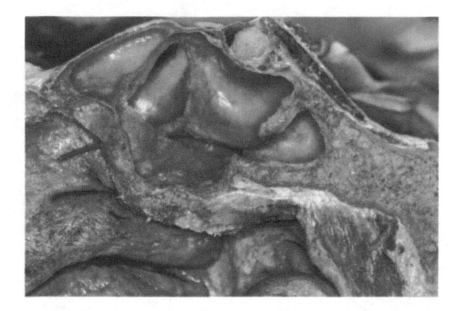

Chapter 10 _____
Sphenoidal Sinus

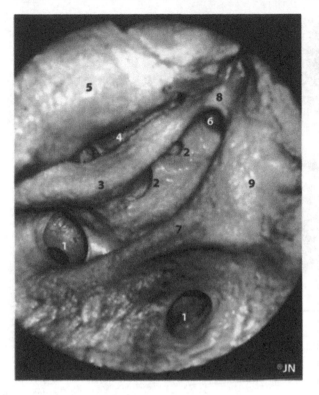

Fig. 129. Detail of the middle nasal meatus, left side

1. accessory ostium of maxillary sinus	5. middle nasal concha (reflected)
2. ostium of anterior ethmoidal cells	6. ostium of frontal sinus
3. ethmoidal bulla	7. uncinate process
4. lateral sinus	8. frontonasal recess
	9. aditus of middle nasal meatus

At the end of the fetal stage, the sites of origin of the future frontal and sphenoidal sinuses in the nasal epithelium display small frontoethmoidal and sphenoethmoidal recesses of a few millimeters, which immediately after birth start to pneumatize these bones. However, these sinuses become radiographically visible only after the fourth year. Due to the characteristics of these bones, their respective sinuses are apt to grow so much within them as to reach large volumes and the most variable shapes.

The ostium of the sphenoidal sinus is about 8–10 mm under the nasal roof, in the superior third of the sphenoethmoidal recess (Fig. 131). In spite of the great anatomical variations of this sinus, its ostium is always in the recess, between the nasal septum and the nasal lateral wall, at the level of the caudal portion of the superior nasal concha.

In the classification proposed by van Alyea, there are three types of sphenoidal sinuses, according to their relation with the hypophysial fossa, namely the conchal, the pre-saddle, and the saddle type. The conchal sinus is restricted to a small anterior (or conchal) region of the body of the sphenoid; the pre-saddle sinus is tangent to the anteri-

or edge of the hypophysial fossa, and the saddle sinus would be under this edge.

The basilar kind of expansion, described by the earliest authors such as Sieur and Jacob and Hajek at the beginning of the twentieth century, is presently regarded not as a sinus on its own, but as a posterior expansion of the saddle-type sinus approaching the basilar surface of the occipital bone, occasionally causing dehiscences in this wall. Such dehiscences are apt to expose the meninges and the occipital venous plexus, creating a connection between the two cavernous sinuses. This kind of sinus is present in as many as 40% of cases; it can be detected by means of axial tomography, especially due to its anatomical relationship with the internal carotid artery.

The expansions and recesses of the sphenoidal sinus are not infrequent and have been extensively described in the literature. The most common type of expansion is one on the sinusal floor, or pterygoidal recess. It involves the canal of the pterygoid nerve (Fig. 129), rendering it dehiscent in the large expansions. The inferolateral prolongation of this sinus gains the interior of the pterygoidal and sphenoidal processes, involving occasionally even the insertion of the medial pterygoid muscle. This is visible on axial tomography as radiolucent circles inside these processes (Figs. 136, 139). The sinusal expansion continues laterally towards the greater wing of the sphenoid, following a pathway under the cavernous sinus, usually not involved by the expansion. However, the round canal for the trigeminal maxillary branch is often totally or partially surrounded by the sinus, which may extend further to the temporal boundaries of the greater wing and eventually emerge in the temporal fossa (Figs. 135–138).

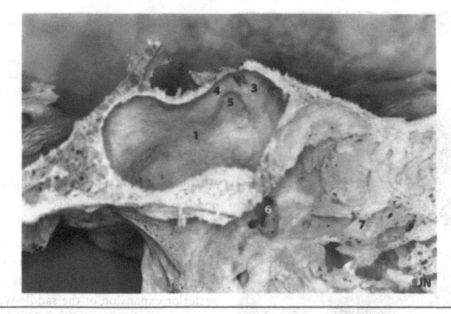

Fig. 130. Left bony sphenoidal sinus, sellar type

1. sphenoidal sinus	3. optic canal prominence	4. carotid prominence	5. carotid-optic recess
2. hypophysial fossa	in the anterosuperior	in the laterosuperior	6. sphenopalatine foramen
	sinusal wall	sinus wall	7. nasal cavity, lateral wall

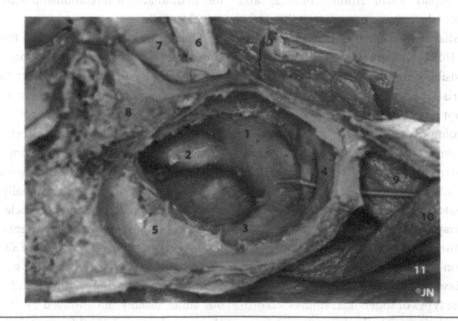

Fig. 131. Left sphenoidal sinus, sellar type

Prominences of:	4. ostium of sphenoidal	6. optic nerve	10. middle nasal concha
1. the optic canal	sinus (green probe)	7. internal carotid artery	(reflected)
2. round canal	5. sphenoidal sinus,	8. hypophysis	11. middle nasal meatus
3. pterygoid nerve canal	main septum (resected)	9. superior nasal concha	

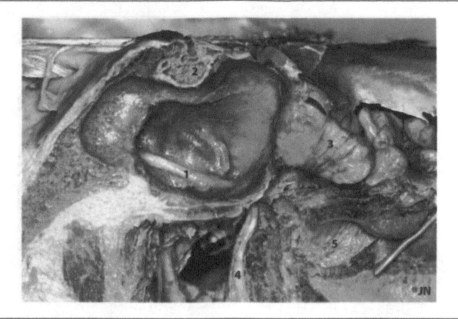

Fig. 132. Left sphenoidal sinus, basilar type

1. prominence of the pterygoid nerve canal on the sinus floor	2. hypophysis 3. posterior ethmoidal cell	4. pterygopalatine fossa	5. nasal cavity, lateral wall

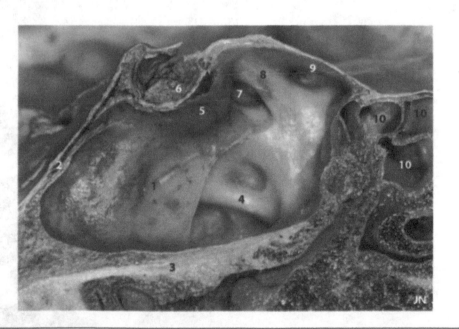

Fig. 133. Left sphenoidal sinus, basilar type

1. sphenoidal sinus, accessory septum 2. basilar wall (posterior) of the sphenoidal sinus 3. sphenoidal sinus floor	4. round canal prominence at the lateral wall of sphenoidal sinus 5. internal carotid artery prominence in the lateral and posterior walls of the sphenoidal sinus	6. pituitary gland in the hypophyseal fossa 7. carotid-optic recess 8. optic canal prominence on laterosuperior wall of sphenoidal sinus	9. sphenoidal sinus expansion into the sphenoidal lesser wing 10. posterior ethmoidal cell

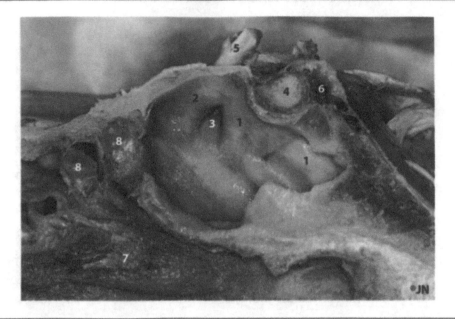

Fig. 134. Right sphenoidal sinus, sellar type

1. prominence of the vertical intracavernous segment of the internal carotid artery at the lateral and posterior sinus walls	2. optic canal salience in the laterosuperior sinus wall	3. carotid-optic recess 4. hypophysis 5. optic nerve	6. basilar venous plexus 7. nasal cavity, lateral wall 8. posterior ethmoidal cell

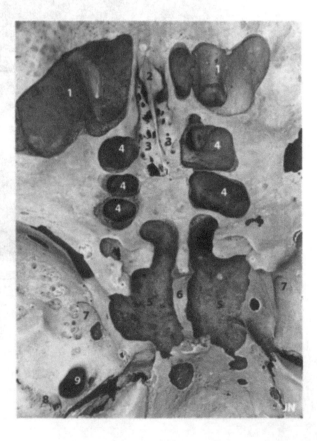

Fig. 135. Cranial view of the bony paranasal sinuses

1. frontal sinus	6. sphenoidal sinus, main septum
2. crista galli	7. round foramen
3. ethmoidal cribriform plate	8. foramen spinosum
4. ethmoidal cell	9. oval foramen
5. sphenoidal sinus	

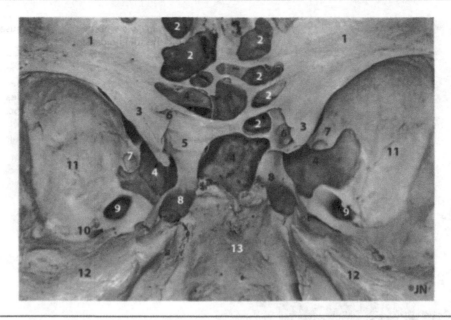

Fig. 136. Cranial view of the bony paranasal sinuses

1. frontal orbital plate	5. septum of sphenoidal	8. carotid groove	12. temporal petrous
2. ethmoidal cell	sinus	9. oval foramen	portion
3. anterior clinoid process	6. optic canal	10. spinosum foramen	13. basilar process
4. sphenoidal sinus	7. round canal	11. middle cranial fossa	

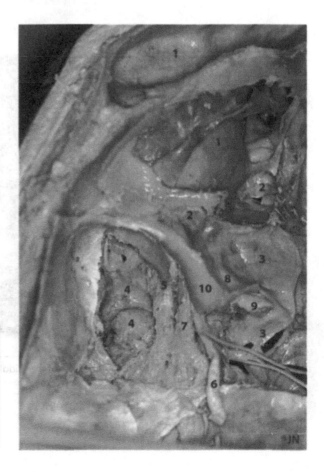

Fig. 137. Cranial view of the paranasal sinuses, left side

1. frontal sinus	6. common ocular motor
2. ethmoidal cell	nerve
3. sphenoidal sinus	7. ophthalmic nerve
4. lateral expansion	8. prominence
of sphenoidal sinus	of the optic canal into
to interior of sphenoid	the sphenoidal sinus
great wing	9. optic nerve
5. maxillary nerve	10. anterior clinoid process

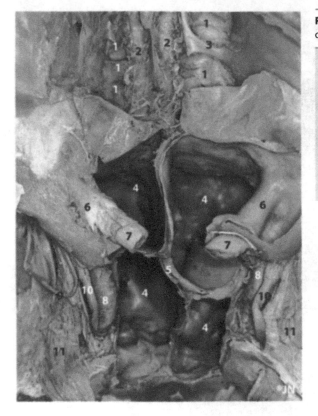

Fig. 138. Cranial view of the paranasal sinuses and the optic canals into the sphenoidal sinuses

1. ethmoidal cell	7. optic nerve
2. ethmoidal cribriform plate	8. internal carotid artery
3. anterior ethmoidal canal	9. trochlear nerve
4. sphenoidal sinus	10. common ocular motor nerve
5. sphenoidal sinus, main septum	11. trigeminal ganglion
6. optic canal, large bilateral prominence into the sphenoidal sinuses	

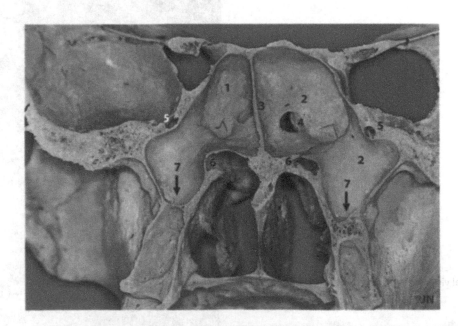

Fig. 139. Coronal section of the cranium at the level of the middle sphenoidal sinus, posterior view

1. left sphenoidal sinus	4. right sphenoidal sinus ostium	6. pterygoid nerve canal region	7. sphenoidal sinus, pterygoid expansion (arrows)
2. right sphenoidal sinus	5. round canal		
3. sphenoidal sinus, main septum			

Although there is little mention in the literature about it, the sphenoidal sinus may occasionally approach the oval foramen (trigeminal mandibular branch) and the foramen spinosum (middle meningeal artery). Accessing the zygomatic region in the presence of such expansions will reveal the sphenoidal sinus to be on the bony base of the middle cranial fossa, over or medial to the lateral pterygoid muscle. Expansions toward the lesser wing of the sphenoid are less frequent, affecting most importantly the optic canal, which may be partly or totally involved (Figs. 133–138). However, even in the absence of such expansions, the optic canal may be related to the sphenoidal sinus, protruding in the laterosuperoanterior walls of small pre-saddle sinuses. The same occurs with the cavernous portion of the internal carotid artery, whose siphon may partly or totally protrude on the posterior and laterosuperior walls of the sphenoidal sinus (Figs. 130, 131, 133, 135). The degree of relationship of these structures with the sinuses is quite variable and is linked to age as well as to racial and genetic factors. However, even reaching great proportions with incredible anatomical variations, the sphenoidal sinus does not invade the cavernous, the hypophysial, or the choanal spaces. A parasagittal accessory bony septum in an oblique position is frequently found, starting from the anterior border of the posterior vertical segment of the bony wall anterior to the internal carotid artery and ending at the middle one third of the sphenoidal sinus (Fig. 130). This is a useful anatomosurgical point of reference, since it is easily identified on axial tomographs of the sinus. In its anterior segment, the internal carotid artery is situated posterior to the optic canal, forming with it a 90° angle and a small recess, termed the carotid-optic recess by Sieur and Jacob early in the twentieth century. This recess harbors several tributary venules supplying the cavernous sinuses (Figs. 133–138).

The sphenoidal sinus and the posterior ethmoidal cells are of anatomosurgical importance due to their proximity to vital structures such as the internal carotid artery, hypophysis, optic nerve, and cavernous sinus (Figs. 133, 134, 136).

Chapter 11
Cranial Base
and Paranasal Sinuses

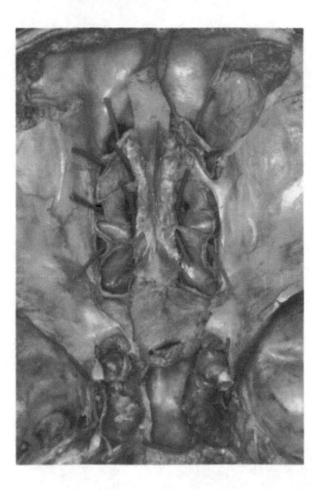

Chapter 11
Cranial Base
and Paranasal Sinuses

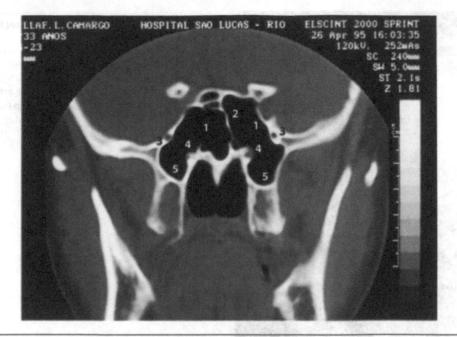

Fig. 140. Coronal CT of an adult, at the level of the middle sphenoidal sinus

1. sphenoidal sinus
2. sphenoidal sinus,
   main septum
	3. round canal
	4. pterygoid nerve canal
		5. sphenoidal sinus,
		   pterygoid expansion
			(Reproduced with thanks to
			Dr. R.M. Neves Pinto,
			Rio de Janeiro, Brazil)

The ethmoidal cells seldom remain contained within the interorbital space. The frontal sinus expands naturally to the interior of the frontal bone, including the interior of its orbital plates. However, the anterior ethmoidal cells do the same, competing for space with the frontal sinus. The sphenoidal sinus grows inside the sphenoid but may also approach the ethmoidal cells and the maxillary sinus (Figs. 140–142).

The ethmoidal cells expand laterally over the orbit and between the orbit and the maxillary sinus (Haller cells). The most diverse anatomical relationships result from this „competition" for space, making the systematization of the sinuses a hard task. With respect to the ethmoidal cells, the anterior ones are generally positioned at the most superior level in the anterior fossa of the cranium. This is due to the presence of the ethmoidal fovea beside and above the cribriform plate of the ethmoid. Distal to the crista galli and the cribriform plate, the posterior ethmoidal cells are situated in a more regular plane, articulating with the lesser wing and with the body of the sphenoid itself. Anteriorly, the greatest anatomosurgical risk is posed by the relationship of the fovea with the cribriform lamina, mainly when the ethmoidal bulla is the fovea. Posteriorly, the risk is present in the relation of the posterior cells with the optic canal (Figs. 143, 149, 150). When the crista galli process is pneumatized by the frontal sinus and the ethmoidal fovea extends over the cribriform lamina, the olfactory fossa is reduced and the olfactory bulbs are compressed (Figs. 145, 146).

The posterior ethmoidal cells and the sphenoidal sinus constantly compete for space. When the posterior cells are voluminous, the sphenoidal sinus is apparently smaller, and vice versa. However, the spatial distribution of these cavities is highly variable (Figs. 144–150).

The posterior ethmoidal cells may occasionally grow so as to cross the median sagittal plane, reaching a position anterior to the sphenoidal sinus, thus reducing or even eliminating the sphenoethmoidal recess.

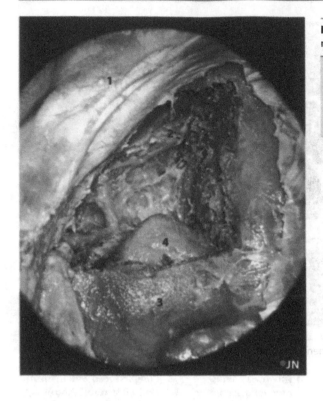

Fig. 141. Inside of the pterygoid process, near the middle cranial fossa, right side

1. sphenoid, lesser wing 2. sphenoid, great wing 3. sphenoidal sinus	4. pterygoid expansion enveloping the medial pterygoid muscle insertion (see axial CT in Fig. 142)

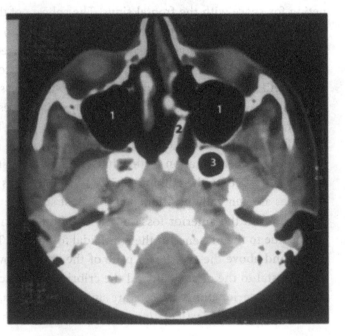

Fig. 142. Axial CT of the nasal cavity and paranasal sinuses

1. maxillary sinus
2. nasal septum
3. sphenoidal sinus, pterygoid expansion

(Reproduced with thanks to Dr. Celso Pita, Hospital Moinho de Vento, Porto Alegre, Brazil)

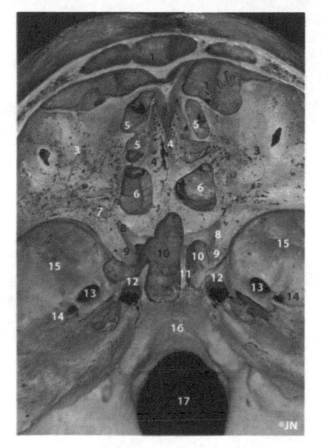

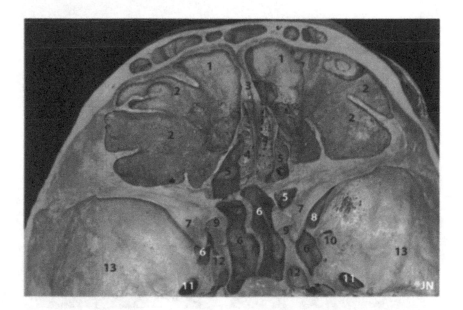

Fig. 143. Cranial view of the bony paranasal sinuses

1. frontal sinus	10. sphenoidal sinus
2. crista galli	11. sphenoidal sinus,
3. frontal orbital plate	main septum
4. ethmoidal cribriform	12. carotid groove
plate	13. oval foramen
5. anterior ethmoidal cells	14. foramen spinosum
6. posterior ethmoidal cells	15. middle cranial fossa
7. sphenoid, lesser wing	16. clivus
8. optic canal	17. foramen magnum
9. anterior clinoid process	

Fig. 144. Cranial view of the bony paranasal sinuses

1. frontal sinus	4. ethmoidal cribriform	7. anterior clinoid process	10. round canal
2. anterior ethmoidal cell	plate	8. superior orbital fissure	11. oval foramen
3. crista galli	5. posterior ethmoidal cell	9. optic canal	12. carotid groove
	6. sphenoidal sinus		13. middle cranial fossa

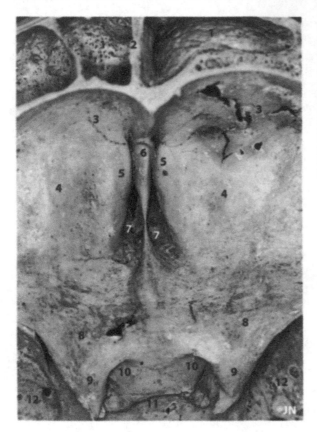

Fig. 145. Bony anterior cranial base and frontal sinuses

1. frontal sinus with anterior ethmoidal cells (frontal bullae)	5. ethmoidal fovea
	6. crista galli
	7. ethmoidal cribriform plate
2. frontal sinus, main septum	8. sphenoid, lesser wing
3. the bone rupture suggests dehiscence of the ethmoidal cell roof	9. anterior clinoid process
	10. optic canal
	11. hypophysial fossa
4. frontal orbital plate	12. middle cranial fossa

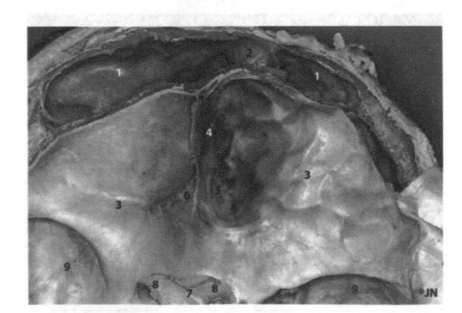

Fig. 146. Anterior cranial base and frontal sinuses

1. frontal sinus	4. crista galli	6. left olfactory fossa reduced by expansion of frontal sinus	7. optic chiasm
2. frontal sinus, main septum	5. ethmoid cribriform plate		8. optic nerve
3. frontal orbital plate			9. middle cranial fossa

By means of a dissection technique similar to that used for the ethmoidal cells via the orbit, the roofs of the ethmoidal cells and of the frontal and sphenoidal sinuses are removed. The frontal sinus and the anterior ethmoidal cells present a very varied anatomical relationship, particularly in their supraorbital expansions. Their cranial aspect is not always representative of their form and volume. Moreover, they may be not detectable from a cranial view, but present elsewhere (Figs. 147, 148).

The posterior and anterior ethmoidal canals may be present among the cells, over them, or under their respective roofs. The anterior ethmoidal canal is more individualized and regular in its course; the posterior one is thinner and sometimes multiple, branching off posterior to the cribriform plate of the ethmoid.

By expanding laterally and posteriorly, the posterior cells may come very close to the optic canal,

leading eventually to its dehiscence. The most frequent is the C-shaped involvement of the optic canal by the cell. The posterior ethmoidal cells tend to occupy the entire space of the superior nasal meatus, protruding into the posterosuperior region of the nasal cavity and obstructing part of the choanae (Figs. 149, 150).

The anatomical relationship of the ethmoidal fovea with the cribriform plate constitutes a high surgical and traumatic risk. The interorbital and supraorbital cellular expansion determine the degree of this relationship. The pneumatization of the crista galli and the medial and posterior expansion of the frontal sinus also add to the risk posed by the presence of the ethmoidal fovea. The cranial aperture of the anterior ethmoidal canal is in this area, at the level of the junction of the fovea with the cribriform plate. The discrepancy in level between the cribriform lamina and the ethmoidal fovea varies from 0 to 25 mm.

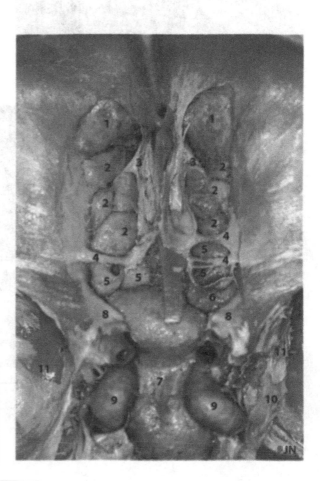

Fig. 147. Cranial view of the paranasal sinuses

1. frontal sinus	7. left sphenoidal sinus
2. anterior ethmoidal cell	8. optic nerve
3. anterior ethmoidal canal	9. internal carotid artery
4. posterior ethmoidal canal	10. trigeminal ganglion
5. posterior ethmoidal cell	11. middle cranial fossa
6. right sphenoidal sinus	

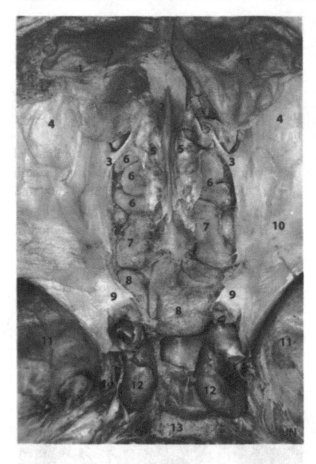

Fig. 148. Cranial view of the paranasal sinuses

1. frontal sinus	7. posterior ethmoidal cell
2. crista galli	8. sphenoidal sinus
3. anterior ethmoidal canal	9. optic nerve
4. anterior ethmoidal cell (supraorbital expansion)	10. anterior cranial fossa
	11. middle cranial fossa
5. ethmoidal cribriform plate	12. internal carotid artery
	13. basilar process of sphenoid
6. anterior ethmoidal cell	

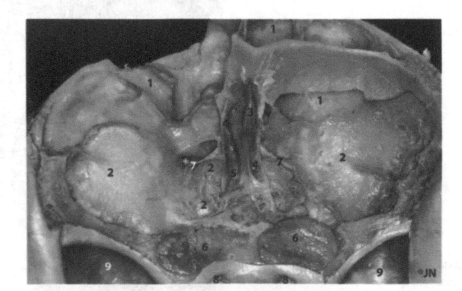

Fig. 149. Cranial view of the paranasal sinuses

1. frontal sinus	3. crista galli	5. posterior ethmoidal artery	8. optic nerve
2. large anterior ethmoidal cell	4. ethmoidal cribriform plate	6. posterior ethmoidal cell	9. middle cranial fossa
		7. anterior ethmoidal canal	

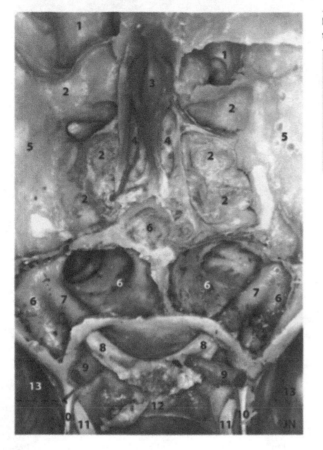

Fig. 150. Cranial view of the paranasal sinuses in relation to the optic nerve

1. frontal sinus	8. optic nerve
2. anterior ethmoidal cell	9. internal carotid artery
3. crista galli	10. trochlear nerve
4. ethmoidal cribriform plate	11. common ocular motor nerve
5. orbit	12. hypophysial fossa
6. posterior ethmoidal cell	13. middle cranial fossa
7. optic canal	

Chapter 12
Notes of Anatomosurgical Importance

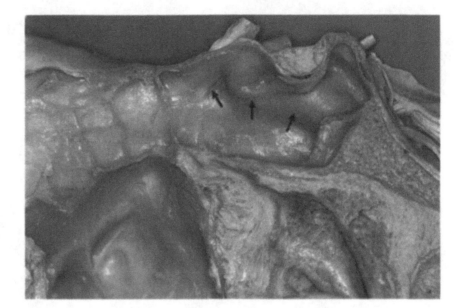

Chapter 12

Notes of Anatomosurgical Importance

1. Nasal Cavity

Pneumatization: • In anterior and posterior segments: 8% – (Grunwald, cited by Lawson, 1964) • Bullar concha (Zuckerkandl 1893)	**Straight septum, in newborn:** • Davis (1914) • Schaeffer (1916)

Deviation of the vomer and cartilage from the median plane in the newborn:
• Neumann (cited by Lawson, 1964)
• 1 case (Patrzek, cited by Lang, 1989)
• Peter (1925)
• Hillenbrand (1923) 93 cases:
  – 36 straight septa (Metzenbaum 1936)
  – 57 vomer asymmetries, inclination, thickening, and cartilage wrinkles
	Septal deviation:
	• In the fetus: two cases (Boyden 1948), one case (Patrzek 1980)
	• In the newborn: 16% (Anton 1893), (Metzenbaum 1936)
	• In the adult: 22% (Theile 1855), 63% (Stier 1895), 75% (McKenzie 1923)
	
	Septal Perforation:
	• 8 of 150 cases – (Zuckerkandl 1893)

Causes of septal deviation (Grunwald): • Uneven growth between the maxillary and palatine septa • Subluxations • Growth of the middle concha • Newborn: changes in the bone pressure	**Septal Pneumatization (by the expansion of the sphenoidal sinus):** • Onodi (1893) • Schaeffer (1920) • Krmpotić and Nemanić (1977) • Lang (1989)
Traumas and absence of septum: • Cartilaginous (Heymann 1900, Melaughlin 1949) • Vomer, perpendicular plate and nasal concha; one case (Lang and Kley 1981)	**The middle nasal concha marks the junction of the roof of the nasal cavity with the ethmoidal labyrinth (Lawson 1964)**

2. Maxillary Sinus

In relation to the floor of the nasal cavity: • At birth – 4 mm above • From 8 to 9 years – same level • In the adult – 4 mm below	• Gruber (1848, 1850) • Yoshinaga (1909)
Relation with the infraorbital canal: • Dehiscence – 14% (Lang and Papke 1984) • Ostium greater than 3 mm (canal) • Ostium – 17%, canal – 83% (Simon 1939) • Complete septum: one case – 2.5%	**Duplication with comunication:** • 6% – (Lang and Papke 1982, 1984) **Number of accessory ostia:** • one ostium – 23% • three ostia – 0.6% • four ostia – 2.81% (van Alyea 1936)

Main ostium of the maxillary sinus:
- Surgically accessible: 54.6%
- Obstructed by the uncinate process (Myerson 1932)
- Canal-shaped (Dintenfass 1932)

Floor of the maxillary sinus and root apices (Harrison 1961):
- Distance ±0.5 mm above the:
  - 1st upper premolar – 5%
  - 2nd upper premolar – 20%
  - 1st upper molar – 27%
  - 2nd upper molar – 46%
  - 3rd upper molar – 30%

Floor of the maxillary sinus:
- At 2–3 years – a little below the articulation of the inferior nasal concha
- At 7 years – at the level of the inferior meatus
- At 9 years – at the level of the nasal floor
- After 9 years
  - below the level of the nasal floor, 26%
  - at the same level, 28%
  - above, 6%

Frequency of accessory ostium:
- Zuckerkandl (1893) – 9.5%
- Lang and Sakals (1982) – 9.5%
- van Alyea (1936) – 23%
- Neivert (1930) – 25%
- Schaeffer (1920) – 43%

Bony septa and fibromucous folds:
- Lang and Papke (1984) – 10%
- Sagittal septum: Abbada (1937)

Location of the main ostium in the semilunar hiatus:
- Posterior end – 23% (Myerson 1932)
- Posterior one fourth – 2% (Lang and Sakals 1982)
- Posterior three fourths – 48%
- Middle one third – 28%
- Anterior one fourth – 22%
- Anterior one third – 5.4% (van Alyea 1936)
- Middle one third – 10.8%
- Posterior one third – 71.8%

Uncinate process (Myerson 1932) – 114 cases
- Absent – 3
- Rudimentary – 10
- Prominent – 69
- Pronounced – 32

Maxillary sinus and teeth (Harrison 1981)
- 1st upper molar – 2.2%
- 2nd upper molar – 2.2%

Recesses of the maxillary sinus:
- Palatine, infraorbital, zygomatic, and alveolar

3. Frontal Sinus

Sites of opening of the frontal sinus in the nasal cavity:
- Infundibulum:
  - 50% – (Schaeffer 1920)
  - 38% – (Kasper 1936)
  - 55% – (van Alyea 1936)
  - 48.4% – (Lang 1989)

- In the frontoethmoidal recess:
  - 62% – (Schaeffer 1920)
  - 30% – (van Alyea 1936)
  - 26.3% – (Lang 1989)
- In front of the semilunar hiatus: 50%
- In its anterior end: 22%
- In its anterior one fourth: 26%
- Above the semilunar hiatus: 2% (Lang and Haas 1988)

- In the frontal recess: 60%
- Above the superior boundary of the infundibulum: 34%
- In the infundibulum: 4%–15% (van Alyea 1936, Kasper 1936)
- In the infundibular region (Killian, cited by Lang, 1989)

Origin of the frontal sinus:
- Direct: in the frontal recess of the ethmoidal infundibulum
- Indirect: expansion of an ethmoidal cell to the frontal bone and recess (Boyer 1905, Killian, cited by Lang, 1989, Peter 1913, Grunwald 1925)

Post-natal growth of the frontal sinus:
- Start: 3.5 years (Onodi 1891)
- Slow up to 11 years and fast thereafter (Szilvassy 1981)
- Adult shape at 20 years (Koch 1980)
- Maximal pneumatization at 40 years (Stern 1939)
- Pneumatization proceeds after 40 years (Finky and Kraft 1992)

Drainage of the frontal sinus:
- Most common: in the frontal recess – 60%
- Above the infundibulum – 34%
- In the infundibulum – 4%
- In the ethmoidal bulla – 2% (Lawson 1964)

4. Ethmoidal Sinus

Structures opening in the ethmoidal infundibulum:
- Duct of the frontal sinus
- Anterosuperior ethmoidal cells
- Frontal and nasal lacrimal cells of the agger nasi

Middle nasal concha pneumatized by ethmoidal cells:
- Anterior – 55%
- Posterior – 45% (Lawson 1964)

The ethmoidal bulla pneumatizes a large part of the ethmoidal labyrinth:
- Anteriorly – infundibulum
- Posteriorly – distal to the posterior cells (near the sphenoidal sinus) Sommering (1809), Zuckerkandl (1893), Grunwald (1925), van Alyea (1939), Lang et al. (1983)

Cribriform foramina in the frontal recess:
- 10% – (Tonndorf, cited by Stupka 1938)

Ethmoidal cell in the frontal sinus:
- Frontal bulla – observed by Zuckerkandl (1893)
  - 8.9% – (Sieur and Jacob 1901)
  - 20% – (Onodi, cited by Lang 1989)
  - 50% – (van Alyea 1941)

Cells related to the main ostium of the maxillary sinus:
- 16.5% – van Alyea (1936)
- 15.3% – Nikolic (1967)
- 17% – Lang and Haas (1988)

Cells in the posterior wall of the maxillary sinus:
- 8% – Prott (1914) and Dixon (1958)

Superomedial wall of an anterior cell bordering the olfactory groove:
- Rarefied – 38%
- Dehiscent – 14% (Onishi 1981)

Haller cells (orbitomaxillary cells):

- Sinusal prominences (Stupka 1938) divide the maxillary sinus in two (Schlungbaum 1921)
- If well-developed they partly separate the orbit from the maxillary sinus (Terrahe and Muendnich 1973).

Medial pneumatization, between the orbit and the maxillary sinus – 4% (Grunwald 1925)
May obstruct cellular and main ostia of the maxillary sinus (Messerklinger, cited by Lang 1989)

Ethmoidal cell and optic canal:

- Wall of the superior canal involved by the cell – 25% (Habal et al. 1976)
- Very thin wall between Onodi cell and the canal (Lang and Haas 1979)

Basal lamella of the ethmoidal labyrinth (Seydel 1891 and Hajek 1909):

- Bone projections of the lateral wall of the nasal cavity medial to the orbit
- Basal portions of the conchae (roots), in their nasal origins

Relationships of the posterior ethmoidal cell and of the sphenoidal sinus (Siebert 1993)

- Posterior ethmoidal cell and optic canal – 57 cases
  - prominence – 16 cases
  - dehiscence – 2 cases
- Sphenoidal sinus and optic canal – 6 cases
- Sphenoidal sinus plus ethmoidal cell plus optic canal – 7.3%

Ethmoidal cribriform plate is below the level of the ethmoidal cells (ethmoidal fovea; Keros 1962):

- 1–3 mm – 12%
- 4–7 mm – 70%
- 8–16 mm – 18%

Number of ethmoidal cells

Reference	Minimum	Maximum	Median
Ranglanet (1895)	5	14	8–9
Sieur and Jacob (1901)	5	13	7–9
Mosher (1929)	3	15	–
van Alyea (1941)	4	17	9
Lawson (1964)	–	–	7–8
Dixon (1958)	2	20	–

Ethmoidal cells project into frontal sinus in 10%–20% of cases (Dixon 1958, Salinger 1965, Lang 1988)

Incidence of agger nasi cells:

- Dissections
  - 10%–15% – Messerklinger (1967)
  - 40% – Mosher (1929)
  - 65% – Davis (1914)
  - 89% – van Alyea (1939)
- Tomography
  - 98.5% – Bolger et al. (1991) (202 cases)
  - 100% – Zinreich et al. (1988)

Pneumatization of the uncinate process:

- Radiographic studies: 0.4% – Zinreich et al. (1988) (230 cases)
- As an extension of the agger nasi: 2.5% – Bolger et al. (1991) (202 cases)

5. Sphenoidal Sinus

Average volume of the three sinus types:
- Saddle 69%, 6.10 ml
- Pre-saddle 6%, 1.90 ml
- Saddle/conchal 5%, 0.58 ml

Frequency of the three sinus types (Hammer and Radberg 1961):
- Saddle (bilateral) – 48%
- Saddle/pre-saddle – 36%
- Saddle/conchal – 6%

Clinical importance of the sphenoidal sinus:
- Appears around the fourth year (Fujioka and Young 1978)
- Resistance to pneumatization provided by crests and accessory septa within the sinuses (Shopfner 1968)
- Reaches adult size at 13–20 years (Leune 1978)

Relationship of the sphenoidal sinus with the optic canal:
- Canal projection – 57%
  - Minor – 22%
  - Moderate – 30%
  - Pronounced – 5%
- Dehiscence – 1%

Clear sphenoethmoidal recess - 48% (Lang and Sakals 1982)

Location of the ostium of the sphenoidal sinus (Lawson 1964):
- Approximately 8 mm below the cribriform lamina
- Approximately 7 cm and 30∞ from the nasal aperture

Types of sphenoidal ostium:
- Round – 70%
- Elliptic – 30%
- Oval – 15%

Relationship of the internal carotid artery with the sphenoidal sinus:
- Thin bony plate – frequent
- Dehiscence – rare

Relationship of the canal of the pterygoid nerve with the floor of the sphenoidal sinus (Lang and Keller 1977):
- Below the floor – 38%
- Same level – 34%
- Above (in the sinus) – 18%

Rudimentary sphenoidal sinuses:
- Absent – 1%–1.5% (Grunwald 1925)
- Small and lateral (Stupka 1938)
- Small, with septum (Lang and Kley 1981)
- Small, agenesis (Peele 1957)

A well-pneumatized sinus may be around the optic nerve (Harrison 1961)

Less-pneumatized sinuses give space to posterior ethmoidal cells (Lawson 1964)

Great proximity to the optic canal (200 cases, Dixon 1958):
- Posterior ethmoid – 4%
- Sphenoidal sinus – 8%

Bony dehiscences in the lateral wall of the sphenoidal sinus, exposing the internal carotid artery:
- 4% – Renn and Rhoton 1975 (28 of 70 cases)
- 8% – Fujii et al. 1979 (2 of 25 cases)
- 22% – Zinreich et al. 1988 (42 of 188 cases)

Cavernous portion of the internal carotid artery was related to the posterior ethmoidal cells in three cases (Lawson 1964)

Relationship of the horizontal portion of the internal carotid artery, in the cavernous sinus, with the sphenoidal sinus:

- 67% – Sieber 1993 (in 57 cases)
- Types:
  - Saddle – 75%
  - Pre-saddle – 54%
- Projection in the sinusal wall:
  - Minor – 36 cases
  - Moderate – 27 cases
  - Pronounced – 4 cases
- Thickness of the bony sinus wall: 0.52 mm (0–1.2 mm)

Relationship of the horizontal portion of the internal carotid artery in the cavernous sinus with the sphenoidal sinus and the posterior ethmoidal cell:

- Arterial dehiscence in the sinus – 6 cases
- Projection in the cell – 6 cases

Table 1. Dimensions of the paranasal sinuses (Onodi)[a]

Age	Sinus	Length (mm)	Height (mm)	Width (mm)
Newborn	Ethmoidal			
	Anterior	1–5	1–3	1–3
	Posterior	2.5–5	4.5–5	1.5–2
	Frontal	3	4.5	2
	Maxillary	2	4	3
	Sphenoidal	2	4	2
1 year	Ethmoidal			
	Anterior	1–9	1–8	1–6
	Posterior	2–10	2–8	1.5–8
	Frontal	3.5–8	3–9	2–6
	Maxillary	5–19	3–9	2–6
	Sphenoidal	1–9	1–5	1–6
1–4 years	Ethmoidal			
	anterior	3–8	3.5–1	13–6
	posterior	3.5–11	3.5–10	3–11
	Frontal	6.5	6	5
	Maxillary	26	13	12
	Sphenoidal	2.5–5	4.5–6	7
4–8 years	Ethmoidal			
	anterior	5–6	8–13	7
	posterior	11–17	6–9	10
	Frontal	4–11	14–17	7–9
	Maxillary	38	23	20
	Sphenoidal	12–13	8–12	11

[a]The data shown in this table represent intervals. Where the interval is not indicated, the measures are identical.

Table 2. Dimensions of the paranasal sinuses (Handerhuber)[a]

Age	Sinus	Length (mm)	Height (mm)	Width (mm)
Newborn	Ethmoidal	8–12	1–5	1–3
	Maxillary	10	4	3
1–4 years	Ethmoidal	12–21	8–16	5–11
	Frontal	4–8	6–9	4–7
	Maxillary	22–30	12–18	11–19
	Sphenoidal	4–6	3–5	6–8
4–8 years	Ethmoidal	18–24	10–15	9–13
	Frontal	6–10	15–16	8–10
	Maxillary	34–38	22–26	18–24
	Sphenoidal	11–14	7–11	9–11

[a]The data shown in this table represent intervals. Where the interval is not indicated, the measures are identical.

Recommended Reading

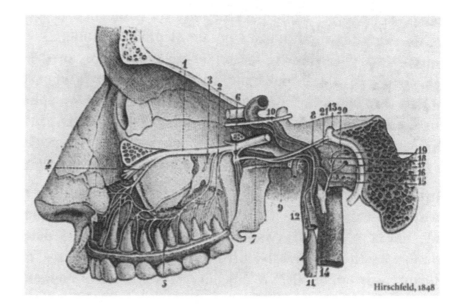

Hirschfeld, 1848

Recommended Reading

Ademà JM, et al (1994) Cirugia endoscopica nasosinusal. Ed.Garsi, Madrid

Almeida CIR (1975) Study of the adenovascular body of the posterior part of the nasal septum. Arch Otolaringol 101: 344–347

Arauz SL (1943) Seno frontal – fisiologia. El Ateneo, Buenos Aires

Bagatella F, Guiraldo CR (1983) The ethmoid labyrinth. An anatomical and radiologic study. Acta Otolaryngol 403 [Suppl]: 1–19

Banberg PS, et al (1987) Relationship of the optic nerve to the paranasal sinuses as shown by computed tomography. Otolaryngol Head Neck Surg 96: 331–335

Becker SP (1989) Anatomy for endoscopic sinus surgery. Otolaryngol Clin North Am 22: 677–682

Becker SP (1994) Applied anatomy of the paranasal sinuses with emphasis on endoscopic surgery, part 2. Ann Otol Rhinol Laryngol 103 [Suppl 162]: 3–32

Blaylock KW, et al (1990) Anterior ethmoid anatomy facilitates dacryocystorhinostomy. Arch Ophthalmol 108: 1774–1777

Blitzer A (1985) Surgery of the paranasal sinuses. Saunders, New York

Bolger WE, et al (1991) Paranasal sinus bony anatomic variations and mucosal abnormalities: CT analysis for endoscopic sinus surgery. Laryngoscope 101: 56–64

Buus DR, et al (1990) Ophthalmic complications of sinus surgery. Ophthalmology 97: 612–619

Calhoun KH, et al (1990) Surgical anatomy of the lateral nasal wall. Otolaryngol Head Neck Surg 102: 156–160

Caliot P, et al (1990) The surgical anatomy of the middle nasal meatus. Surg Radiol Anat 12: 97–101

Caliot JL, et al (1995) The intraorbital arrangement of the anterior and posterior ethmoidal foramina. Surg Radiol Anat 17: 29–33

Canuyt G, Terracol J (1925) Le sinus sphénoidal. Masson, Paris

Clark ST, et al (1989) The incidence of concha bullosa and its relationship to chronic sinonasal disease. Am J Rhinol 3: 11–12

Davis WB (1914) Nasal accessory sinus in man. Saunders, Philadelphia

Dixon FN (1937) A comparative study of the sphenoid sinus (a study of 1600 skulls). Ann Otol Rhinol Laryngol 46: 687–698

Dixon FN (1958) The clinical significance of anatomical arrangement of the paranasal sinus. Ann Otol Rhinol Laryngol 57: 736–741

Dixon HS (1983) Microscopic sinus surgery, transnasal ethmoidectomy and sphenoidectomy and sphenoidectomy. Laryngoscope 93: 440–444

Draf W (1983) Endoscopy of the paranasal sinus. Springer, Berlin Heidelberg New York

Ducasse A, et al (1985) Anatomical basis of the surgical approach to the medial wall of the orbit. Anat Clin 7: 15–21

Duvoisin B, et al (1990) CT study of the ethmoid labyrinth: technique of examination and normal anatomy. Radiol Bras 23: 143–149

Figun ME, Garino RR (1989) Anatomia odontologica funcional e aplicada, 2nd edn. Panamericana, São Paulo

Fireman SM (1976) Dental anatomy and radiology and the maxillary sinus. Otolaryngol Clin North Am 1: 83–91

Fujii K, Chambers SM, Rhoton AL jr (1979) Neurovascular relationships of the sphenoid sinus: a microsurgical study. J Neurosurg 50: 31–39

Habal MB, et al (1976) Microsurgical anatomy of the optic canal: anatomical relations and exposure of the optic nerve. Surg Forum 27: 542–544

Habal MB, Maniscalco JE, Rhoton AL jr (1977) Microsurgical anatomy of the optic canal: correlates to optic nerve exposure. J Surg Res 22: 5527–5533

Hajek M, Heitger AB, Hansel FK (1926) Pathology and treatment of the inflammatory diseases of the nasal accessory sinuses, vol 1. Mosby, St. Louis

Hammer G, Radberg C (1961) The sphenoidal sinus. Acta Radiol 56: 401–422

Hirschfeld P (1866) Traité de l'iconographie de le systeme nerveux et des organes des sens de l'homme, 2nd edn. Masson, Paris

Jovanovic S (1961) Supernumerary frontal sinuses on the roof of the orbit. Acta Anat 45: 133–142

Kainz J, Stammberger H (1989) The roof of the anterior ethmoid: a place of least resistance in the skull base. Am J Rhinol 3: 191–199

Kasper KA (1936) Nasofrontal connections. Arch Otolaryngol 23: 322–343

Killian G (1904) The accessory sinuses of the nose and their relations to neighboring parts. W.T. Keener & Co., Chicago

Kinmann J (1977) Surgical aspects of the sphenoidal sinuses and the sella tursica. J Anat 124: 541–553

Lang J (1989) Clinical anatomy of the nose, nasal cavity, and paranasal sinuses. Thieme, New York

Lang J, Bressel S, Pahnke J (1988) Sphenoidal sinus, clinical anatomy of the approaches to the hypophyseal region. Gegenbaurs Morphologisches Jahrbuch 134: 291–307

Lawson W (1994) The intranasal ethmoidectomy: evolution and an assessment of the procedure. Laryngoscope 104 [Suppl]: 64

Lazorthes G (1955) Le système nerveux périphérique. Masson, Paris

Lofgren RH (1971) Surgery of the pterygomaxillary fossa. Arch Otolaryngol 94: 516–524

Lothrop HA (1903) The anatomy of the inferior ethmoidal turbinate bone with particular reference to cell formation: surgical importance of such ethmoid cells. Ann Surg 38: 233–255

Maniglia AJ (1991) Fatal and other major complications of endoscopic sinus surgery. Laryngoscope 101: 349–354

Manisalco JE, Habal MB (1978) Microanatomy of the optic canal. J Neurosurg 48: 402–406

Masala W, et al (1989) Multiplanar reconstrucions in the study of ethmoid anatomy. Neuroradiology 31: 151–155

Mattox DE, et al (1985) Anatomy of the ethmoid sinus. Otol Clin North Am 18: 3–14

McDonnell D, Esposito M, Todd ME (1992) A teaching model to illustrate the variation in size and shape of the maxillary sinus. J Anat 181: 377–380

Meloni F, et al (1992) Anatomic variations of surgical importance in ethmoid labyrinth and sphenoid sinus. A study of radiological anatomy. Surg Radiol Anat 14: 65–70

Messerklinger W (1967) On the drainage of the normal frontal sinus of man. Acta Otolaryngol 63: 176–181

Messerklinger W (1978) Endoscopy of the nose. Urban & Schwarzenberg, Baltimore

Mocellin L (1964) Um caso de pan agebesia dos seios paranasais. Rev Bras Cir 48: 283–287

Montgomery WW, et al (1970) Analysis of pterygopalatine space surgery. Laryngoscope 80: 1190–1200

Morton EM (1983) Excessive pneumatization of the sphenoid sinus: a case report. J Maxillofac Surg 11: 236–238

Mosher HP (1929) Symposium of the ethmoid. The surgery anatomy of the ethmoid labyrinth. Trans Am Acad Ophthalmol Otolaryngol 34: 376–410

Mosher HP (1929) The surgical anatomy of the ethmoidal labyrinth. Ann Otol Rhinol Laryngol 18: 870–901

Myerson MC (1932) The natural orifice of the maxillary sinus. I. Anatomic studies. Arch Otolaryngol 15: 80–91

Neves-Pinto RM, de Farias UP (1977) Imperfuração coanal congênita e síndrome de Apert. Rev Bras Otorinol 43: 121–126

Neves-Pinto RM, Lima PE (1984) Complicações orbitárias, cranianas e endocranianas das sinusites. F Med (BR) 89: 389–398

Neves-Pinto RM, et al (1996) Tomografia computa-dorizada das cavidades naso-sinusais: algumas ocorrências interessantes. F Med (BR) 112 [Suppl 3]: 225–235

Ohnishi T, et al (1993) High-risk areas in endoscopic sinus surgery and prevention of complications. Laryngoscope 103

Ohnishi T (1981) Bony defects and dehiscences of the roof of the ethmoid cells. Rhinology 19: 195–202

Ohnishi T, et al (1990) Endoscopic microsurgery of the ethmoid sinus. Am J Rhinol 4: 119–127

Onodi A (1895) The anatomy of the nasal cavity and its accessory sinuses: an atlas for students and practioners. Lewis, London

Onodi A (1908) The optic nerve and the accessory cavities of the nose. Contribution to the study of canicular and atrophy of the optic nerves of nasal origin. Ann Otol Rhinol Laryngol 17: 1–116

Prades JM, Veyret CH, Martin CH (1993) Microsurgical anatomy of the ethmoid. Surg Radiol Anat 15: 9–14

Proctor DF (1966) The nose, paranasal sinuses and pharynx. In: Walters W (ed) Lewis-Walters practice of surgery, vol 4. W.F. Prior, Hagerstown, pp 1–37

Rabischong P, et al (1980) Bases anatomiques de l'abord de la fosse pterygopalatine. Anat Clin 2: 209–222

Radoievitch S, Jovanovitch S (1955) La morphologie du canal vidien et ses rapports aveo les sinus paranasaux chez l'homme adulte et l'enfant. Rev Laryngol Otol Rhinol (Bord) 76: 481–492

Radoievitch S, Jovanovitch S (1960) Relations of the optic canal to the posterior paranasal sinuses. Acta Anat 41: 172–183

Renn WH, Rhoton AL (1975) Microsurgical anatomical anatomy of the sellar region. J Neurosurg 43: 288–298

Rice D, Schaefer S (1988) Endoscopic paranasal sinus surgery. Raven, New York

Rice DH (1989) Basic surgical techniques and variations of endoscopic sinus surgery. Otolaryngol Clin North Am 22: 713–726

Ritter FN (1982) The middle turbinate and its relationship to the orbit. Laryngoscope 97: 479–482

Ritter FN (1978) The paranasal sinuses: anatomy and surgical technique. Mosby, St. Louis

Rontal M, Rontal E (1991) Studying whole-mounted sections of the paranasal sinuses to understand the complications of endoscopic sinus surgery. Laryngoscope 101

Rosenberger HC (1938) Clinical availability of ostium maxillare: clinical and cadaver study. Ann Otol Rhinol Laryngol 47:176–182

Rouvière H (1932) Anatomie humaine, 3rd edn. Masson, Paris

Schaeffer JP (1910) On the genesis of air cells in the conchae nasales. Anat Rec 4: 167–180

Schaeffer JP (1910) The sinus maxillaris and its relations in the embryo, child and adult man. Am J Anat 10: 313–368

Schaeffer JP (1916) The genesis, development, and adult anatomy of the nasofrontal region in man. Am J Anat 20: 125–146

Schaeffer JP (1920) The nose, paranasal sinuses, nasolacrimal passageways, and olfactory organ in man. Blakiston, Philadelphia

Schaeffer JP (1942) Morris' human anatomy, 11th edn. McGraw-Hill, London

Shambaugh GE (1907) The construction of the ethmoid labyrinth. Ann Otol Rhinol Laryngol 16: 771–775

Shankar L, et al (1994) An atlas of imaging of the paranasal sinuses. Martin Dunitiz, Singapore

Siebert DR (1994) Anatomia dos seios esfenoidais. Rev Bras Otorrinolaringol 60

Sieur C, Jacob O (1901) Recherches anatomiques, cliniques et opératoires sur les fosses nasales et leurs sinus. Rueff, Paris

Simonetti G, et al (1987) Computed tomography of the ethmoid labyrinth and adjacent structures. Ann Otol Rhinol Laryngol 96: 239–249

Skillern RH (1939) The accessory sinuses of the nose. Lippincott, Philadelphia

Soares M (1980) Anatomia funcional e cirúrgica do nariz. Rev Bras Cir 70: 247–254

Som PM (1985) CT of the paranasal sinuses. Neuroradiology 27: 189–201

Stamm AC, Levon MN, Claudia FP (1988) Microcirurgia transnasal no tratamento da atresia coanal. Rev Bras Otorrinolaringol 54

Stamm AC (1994) Microcirurgia naso-sinusal. Revinter, Rio de Janeiro

Stammberger H (1986) Endoscopic endonasal surgery – concepts in treatment of recurring rhinosinusitis. I. Anatomic and pathophysiologic considerations. Otolaryngol Head Neck Surg 94: 143–147

Stammberger H (1986) Nasal and paranasal sinus endoscopy. A diagnostic and surgical approach to recurrent sinusitis. Endoscopy 18: 213–218

Stammberger H (1989) History of rhinology: anatomy of the paranasal sinuses. Rhinology 27: 197–210

Stammberger H (1991) Functional endoscopic sinus surgery. BC Decker, Philadelphia

Takahashi R (1971) Clinical anatomical studies of the canalis orbitocranialis and canalis orbitoethmoidalis in relation the ethmoid cells. In: Takahashi R (ed) A collection of ear, nose and throat studies. Kyoya, Tokyo

Takahashi R (1983) The formation of the human paranasal sinuses. Acta Otolaryngol [Suppl] 408

Teatini G, et al (1987) Computed tomography of the ethmoid labyrinth and adjacent structures. Ann Otol Rhinol Laryngol 96: 239–250

Terracol J, Ardouin P (1965) Anatomie des fosses nasales et des cavites annexes. Maloine, Paris

Terrier G (1991) Rhinosinusal endoscopy. Diagnosis and surgery. Zambon Group, Milano

Terrier G, et al (1985) Anatomy of the ethmoid: CT, endoscopic, and macroscopic. AJR 144: 493–500

Testut L, Latarjet A (1959) Tratado de anatomia humana, vol 3. Salvat, Barcelona

van Alyea OE (1936) The ostium maxillare: anatomic study of its surgical accessibility. Arch Otolaryngol 24: 553–569

van Alyea OE (1939) Ethmoid labyrinth. Arch Otolaryngol 29: 881–902

van Alyea OE (1941) Sphenoid sinus: anatomic study with considerations of the clinical significance of the structural characteristics of the sphenoid sinus. Arch Otolaryngol 34: 225–253

van Alyea OE (1946) Frontal sinus drainage. Ann Otolaryngol 55: 267–277

van Alyea OE (1951) Nasal sinuses: an anatomic and clinical consideration. Williams and Wilkins, Baltimore

Vidic B (1968) The postnatal development of the sphenoidal sinus and its spread into the dorsum sellae and posterior clinoid process. Am J Roentgenology 104: 177–183

Vidic SB (1969) Extreme development of the paranasal sinuses. Ann Otol 78: 1291–1298

Wallace R, Salazar JE, Cowles S (1990) The relationship between frontal sinus drainage and ostiomeatal complex disease. A CT study on 217 patients. AJNR 11: 183–186

Weiglein A, et al (1992) Radiological anatomy of the paranasal sinuses in the child. Surg Radiol Anat 14: 335–339

Weisman RA (1988) Surgical anatomy of the orbit. Otolaryngol Clin North Am 21: 1–13

Wigand ME (1981) Transnasal ethmoidectomy under endoscopic control. Rhinology 19: 7–15

Wigand ME (1990) Endoscopic surgery of the paranasal sinuses and anterior skull base. Thieme, New York

Zinreich SJ, et al (1987) Paranasal sinuses: CT imaging requirements for endoscopic surgery. Radiology 163: 769–775

Zinreich SJ, et al (1988) Concha bullosa: CT evaluation. J. Comput. Assist. Tomogr 12: 778–784

Zinreich SJ, Kennedy DW, Gayler BW (1988) Computer tomography of nasal cavity and paranasal sinuses: an evaluation of anatomy for endoscopic sinus surgery. Clear Images 1: 2–10

Zuckerkandl E (1895) Anatomie normale et pathologique des fosses nasales et de leurs annexes pneumatiques, vol 2. Masson, Paris

Subject Index

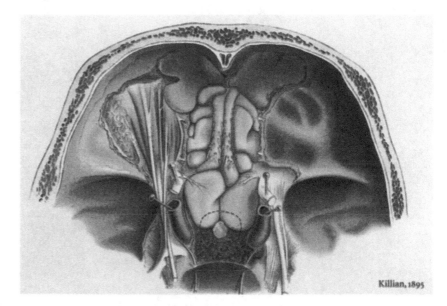

Killian, 1895

Subject Index

A

Aditus 30
- middle nasal meatus 44
Agger nasi 7, 16, 39, 40, 41, 43, 46, 52, 73, 87, 100, 102, 130
Artery
- ethmoidal 4
-- anterior 64, 68
-- posterior 64, 67, 68
- external carotid 63
- facial 64, 68
- internal carotid 63, 113, 114, 131
-- cavernous portion 113
- incisive 64
- infraorbital 76
- maxillary 63, 68, 76, 99
- middle meningeal 107
- nasopalatine 63, 68
- ophthalmic 63, 67, 97
- palatine 68
- posterior lateral nasal 63, 64, 66
- septal 63, 64, 68
Auditory tube 4, 46, 52

B

Basal lamella 40, 95, 97
Basal plate 14
Branchial arch 3
Bulla
- ethmoidal (see Ethmoidal bulla)

C

Canal
- ethmoidal 121
-- anterior 67, 99, 121
-- posterior 121
- frontal sinus 87
- infraorbital 74, 75
- maxillary sinus 64, 99, 113
- optic 113, 117, 121, 130, 131
- pterygoid 107, 113
- round 107
Capsule
- nasal 14
- nasal cartilaginous 14
Carotid-optic 113
Carotid groove 73
Cavernous sinus 113, 131
Choana 33, 43
Choanal region, 46, 47, 52, 58, 75, 87, 102
Concha 40
- bullous 30, 51, 52, 99
- inferior nasal 4, 30, 47, 99, 100
- middle nasal 30, 40, 46, 96, 97, 99,
- nasal 27, 30, 33, 40, 41, 43, 46, 47, 52, 63, 64, 73, 88, 95, 97,
  99, 100, 102, 127, 129
- superior nasal 33, 52, 100
- supreme nasal 40, 52
Crista galli 17, 52, 57, 87, 121, 122

D

Duct
- nasolacrimal 4, 39, 40, 47, 73, 74, 87

E

Ethmoid 4, 27, 39, 64, 85
- cribriform plate 4, 7, 16, 17, 40, 41, 52, 57, 67, 68, 70, 87, 96,
  99, 100, 117, 121, 130
Ethmoidal bulla 7, 28, 33, 39, 40, 44, 46, 47, 52, 73, 74, 87, 96,
  99, 100, 102, 105, 107, 117, 121, 129
Ethmoidal canal
- anterior 67, 99, 121
- posterior 67, 121
Ethmoidal cell 7, 16, 52, 67, 85, 87, 96, 100, 117, 121, 130
- anterior 7, 30, 41, 44, 46, 47, 52, 68, 74, 85, 88, 96, 97, 99,
  100, 105, 121, 130
- posterior 33, 52, 63, 68, 73, 100, 102, 113, 117, 121, 130
- bullous 88
- Onodi 33
- orbitomaxillary 52, 82, 95, 129
Ethmoidal fovea 42, 67, 87, 96, 117, 121
Ethmoido-septal plexus 64
Expansion
- sphenoidal sinus, antero-posterior 74
- sphenoidal sinus, pterygoid 109
External nose 27

F

Foramen
- cribriform 68
- ethmoidal (see Canal, ethmoidal)
- olfactory 68
- optic 67
- oval 107
- round 107
- sphenopalatine 40, 41, 44, 63, 64, 97
- spinous 107, 113
Fossa
- anterior cranial 67, 68
- hypophyseal 104, 107
- middle cranial 107
- pterygopalatine 40, 42, 66, 67, 73, 99
Frontal
- bone 14, 64, 117
- process 7
- recess 7
- sinus 44, 85, 87, 88, 100, 117, 121, 128, 129

G

Ganglion
- pterygopalatine 63, 64
- trigeminal 121
Gland
- hypophysis 113

H

Hiatus
- semilunar (see Semilunar hiatus)

I

Incisive canal 64
Infundibulum 7, 14, 28, 40, 44, 46, 47, 74, 87, 102, 128, 129

L

Lacrimal 39
Lacrimal sac 40, 41, 88

M

Maxillary
– artery 63, 76, 99
– nerve 63, 64, 66
– process
– alveolar 27
–– frontal 27, 39, 40, 43, 47, 87, 95, 102
sinus 14, 16, 27, 30, 39, 43, 46, 47, 52, 63, 73, 74, 75, 76, 95, 99,
　100, 102, 105, 117, 121, 127, 128, 129
Maxillopalatine junction 40, 73
Meatus
– common nasal 30
– inferior nasal 7, 30
– middle nasal 6, 30, 39, 46, 47, 73, 99, 100
– superior nasal 30, 43, 52, 64

N

Nasal 10, 39
– floor 39, 57, 64
– roof 33, 46, 64
Nasal cavity 3, 14, 27, 33 ,39, 40, 41, 46, 52, 57, 60, 63, 64, 66,
　68, 70, 73, 74, 82, 88, 95, 99, 100, 102, 121, 127, 130
Nasal limen 27, 41, 46, 52, 102
Nasal meatus
– middle 7, 16, 30, 39, 46, 47, 73, 99, 100
– common 7, 27
– inferior 7, 30
– superior 30, 43, 52, 64, 99
Nasal septum 14, 27, 87, 88
– cartilaginous portion 57
–– sphenoidal extension 57
Nasal spine
– anterior 27
– posterior 33
Nerve
– maxillary 63, 64
– nasopalatine 68
– optic 68, 96, 97, 113, 121, 131
– ophthalmic 63
– trigeminal 63
Neurocranium 3

O

Olfactory epithelium 4
Olfactory fossa 4
Olfactory mucosa 60
Opening
– anterior ethmoidal cells 41
– nasal 27, 47, 74, 85
– piriform 27, 39, 75
Ophthalmic
– artery and nerve 97

Orbit 16, 95, 99
Orbital
– inferior fissure 63, 64, 86
– superior fissure 29, 86, 95
Orbitomaxillary cells (Haller) 82, 95, 130
Ostium
– cellular 46
– drainage 73, 85
– ethmoidal 88, 102
– frontonasal 85
– maxillary sinus'
–– accesory 14, 16, 100, 102, 128
–– main 73, 79, 99, 100, 102, 128, 129
– sphenoidal 107, 131

P

Palatine 39, 40
Periorbit 67
Piriform aperture 27
Pituitary gland 60
Plate
– cribriform (see Cribriform plate)
– ethmoidal perpendicular 27, 57, 58, 68
– orbital 119
– palatine horizontal 33, 39
– palatine vertical 33, 39, 40, 41, 64
– papirace 95
– pterygoid process, middle 33, 39, 40, 41
Process
– crista galli (see Crista galli, process)
– frontal 27, 30, 39, 40, 46, 47, 86, 95, 102
– maxillary frontal 40, 46, 47
– palatine orbital 95, 99
– pterygoid 39, 40, 41
– uncinate 7, 39, 40, 41, 46, 47, 52, 73, 74, 99, 100, 102, 128, 130
Pterygomaxillary fissure 64
Pterygopalatine fossa 40, 46, 63, 64, 73, 74
Pterygopalatine ganglion 63

R

Recess
– frontal 7
– frontoethmoidal 41, 46, 52, 87, 100, 102, 107, 128
– fronto-nasal 105
– maxillary sinus 75
– spheno-ethmoidal 40, 46, 47, 52, 102, 121, 131
– suprabullar 46, 47
Region
– choanal 46, 47, 52, 58, 75, 88, 102
– nasopharynx 64
– orbitomaxillary 99
– periorbitary 95
– prebullar 87
Roof
– maxillary sinus 73
– nasal 33, 46, 64

S

Septal deviation 30, 127
Semilunar hiatus 7, 40, 41, 46, 47, 88, 102, 128

Septum
- accessory 87
- cartilage 33
- nasal 4, 27, 30, 34, 39, 46, 43, 52, 57, 60, 63, 64, 68, 88, 99, 100
- main bony 87
Sinus
- basilar 113
- cavernous 107, 113, 131
- conchal 113
- ethmoidal 95, 129
- frontal 10, 44, 85, 88, 95, 102, 121
- frontomaxillary 82
- lateral 14, 41, 46, 47, 100, 102, 105
- maxillary 7, 14, 17, 34, 46, 47, 52, 63, 73, 74, 75, 76, 95, 99, 100, 102, 105, 121, 127, 128, 129
- paranasal 3, 67, 85, 95, 99, 100, 132, 133
- presellar 113
- sphenoidal (see Sphenoidal sinus)
Sphenoethmoidal 100, 113, 132
Sphenopalatine foramen 39, 40, 42, 46, 63, 64, 66, 96, 97
Sphenoid 4, 17, 33, 39, 117
Sphenoidal
great wing 14, 107, 110
lesser wing 4, 14, 110
ostium 107, 131
- sinus 14, 16, 17, 39, 40, 41, 46, 52, 57, 63, 68, 73, 74, 75, 95, 99, 100, 102, 107, 113, 115, 117, 119, 121, 127, 129, 131, 132
Spine
- anterior nasal 27
- posterior nasal 33, 39

Suture
- intermaxillary 27
- metopic 85
Synchondrosis 17

U
Uncinate process 14, 16, 39, 40, 44, 46, 47, 52, 66, 73, 74, 99, 100, 102, 105, 128, 130

V
Viscerocranium 3
Vomer 27, 57
- wing 36

W
Wall
- maxillary sinus, anterior 75
- nasal fossa, lateral 73
- maxillary sinus, middle 73
- maxillary sinus, posterior 73, 76
Window
- maxillary anterior 39, 40, 41
- maxillary posterior 39, 40, 41
Wing
- vomer 33
- sphenoidal great 113
- sphenoidal lesser 14, 113